INSTITUTIONALIZING THE INSANE IN NINETEENTH-CENTURY ENGLAND

STUDIES FOR THE SOCIETY FOR THE SOCIAL HISTORY OF MEDICINE

Series Editors: David Cantor
Keir Waddington

TITLES IN THIS SERIES

Forthcoming Titles

www.pickeringchatto.com/sshm

INSTITUTIONALIZING THE INSANE IN NINETEENTH-CENTURY ENGLAND

BY

Anna Shepherd

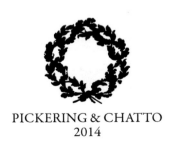

PICKERING & CHATTO
2014

Published by Pickering & Chatto (Publishers) Limited
21 Bloomsbury Way, London WC1A 2TH

2252 Ridge Road, Brookfield, Vermont 05036-9704, USA

www.pickeringchatto.com

BRITISH LIBRARY CATALOGUING IN PUBLICATION DATA

Shepherd, Anna, author.
Institutionalizing the insane in nineteenth-century England. – (Studies for the
Society for the Social History of Medicine)
1. Psychiatric hospital care – England – History – 19th century – Case studies.
I. Title II. Series
362.2'1'0942'09034-dc23

ISBN-13: 9781848934313
e: 9781781440568

This publication is printed on acid-free paper that conforms to the American
National Standard for the Permanence of Paper for Printed Library Materials.

Typeset by Pickering & Chatto (Publishers) Limited
Printed and bound in the United Kingdom by CPI Books

CONTENTS

ACKNOWLEDGEMENTS

I am deeply indebted to the Wellcome Trust for the doctoral studentship that supported my PhD which prompted this study. Many people helped and supported me during the course of my research and the writing of this book. They are too numerous to mention individually and I apologize for not doing so. It would have been impossible for me to have succeeded without their co-operation and assistance.

I was fortunate in that the bulk of the archival material was held in the Surrey History Centre, Woking, where the staff unstintingly gave their time, expertise and every possible assistance, which made my many hours spent there a productive and pleasurable experience. I should particularly like to thank Julian Pooley for his friendship, sense of humour, extensive knowledge and chocolate biscuits during my visits.

I should also like to extend my gratitude to the librarians and archivists at the Wellcome Institute, the National Archives, the Royal Holloway Archives, and the members of staff at the unique Egham Museum. I am particularly grateful to the delightful Joy Whitfield, who shared her experiences and knowledge of the Holloway Sanatorium where she had worked for many years. I would particularly like to thank the staff at the School of Humanities at Oxford Brookes University; Carol Beadle deserves a special mention.

I am also very grateful to Dorothy Porter, who began the journey with me, and Jonathan Andrews, who encouraged me to return to my research following some particularly difficult personal challenges. Anne Digby was my mentor and never ceased to believe in me, to provide advice, constructive criticism and encouragement. A great many friends have supported me in a myriad of ways and I would like to thank them all profusely. Andrea Tanner ceaselessly offered advice and encouragement at every stage, especially when life threatened to intervene and I was ready to submit to the pressures. Graham Mooney has tirelessly supported and encouraged my endeavours, providing constructive insights. David Wight has been a long-standing supporter of my research and been an inspiration since my earliest forages in the archives. Keir Waddington has provided both stick and carrot in equal measure to help me get to this stage; thank you. Last but not least, I want to thank my friends and family for their long-suffering support, but especially my sons, Dominic and Christian Shepherd, who spent some childhood Sundays visiting old asylums with me, and to whom I dedicate this book, with love.

LIST OF FIGURES AND TABLES

INTRODUCTION: CONTEXTS OF INSANITY

Nineteenth-century England witnessed an explosion in the provision of institutionalized care for the insane. The large asylum population was often attributed to the accumulation of chronic patients, who had been admitted with long-established mental illness, the duration of which minimized their chances of recovery. Equally, the poor physical condition of incoming patients had an adverse effect on successful outcomes, and this resulted in pessimism and low expectations amongst the medical staff, particularly in the large county asylums, so that minimal treatment was offered. However, the enduring image of the county asylum as a place of containment and fear has been questioned and efforts made to place the asylum within the broader social context. This has led to considerations of the role of the family in both the incarceration and discharge processes. There has also been increased appreciation of the role of rigid class distinctions in the mental patient experience in both the pauper and private asylum. Official records, whilst valuable, can offer only a limited perspective, so that the reality of the asylum patient experience in the nineteenth century necessarily remains elusive.

By contrasting two geographically close, but ideologically distinct, institutions for the insane in Surrey, *Institutionalizing the Insane* compares the psychiatric care of men and women within the pauper Brookwood Asylum and the Holloway Sanatorium. The rationale behind their establishment suggests that contemporary class perceptions shaped their existence and management. Class defined committal and discharge processes and, combined with contemporary expectations of appropriate behaviour for men and women, influenced diagnosis, treatment and outcomes. Nineteenth-century Surrey was an ideal location for large institutions. Land was cheap, and there were good rail communications, particularly to London. Brookwood Asylum was the county's second public asylum for pauper patients; the first, Springfield, opened in Wandsworth in 1841 and was full to capacity by 1854. Described as 'a cheery hamlet of almshouses', and located on a prime 150-acre site near Woking, Brookwood opened its doors on 17 June 1867.[1] Less than 10 miles away, the privately endowed Holloway Sanatorium was established specifically for the middle-class insane, who had been largely excluded from access to appropriate, and affordable, institutional psychiatric care. It attracted considerable press interest at its official opening by the Prince of Wales on 15 June 1885. Despite the original intention to care solely for middle-class patients, finances dictated that wealthier upper-class men and women were soon being admitted.

A rich scholarship has already explored themes such as the professionalization of treating madness, notions of social control and the role of the state and the impact of legislation on patient care. Debates on the value of institutional regulation of deviance and the difficulty in managing psychiatric patients within the community have prompted a reconsideration of the inherited asylum-centred system.[2] The focus on nineteenth-century mental illness stems from the development of primarily custodial psychiatric care, although studies of earlier psychiatric practices have contributed significantly towards the social history of insanity. The importance of Michel Foucault's contributions to the debate has been acknowledged; although his theory of the 'great confinement' and his neglect of discussions on asylum location and reform can be criticized, his assessment of the impact of the asylum in Western civilization remains highly influential.[3] Since Foucault tended to merge histories of many societies into one chronology, and focused on a few key actors, critics see a distorted perspective of the institution in his work, with the underrating of factors such as social class, family, local networks and politics in the treatment of insanity. More recent scholarship has highlighted the asylum's multiple functions within both varied and specific locations.[4]

These debates paved the way for Andrew Scull's controversial studies which initially focused on the growth of 'asylumdom' in nineteenth-century England. He firstly examined the asylum against a backdrop of a rapidly urbanizing England, where social and familial ties deteriorated. This, he claimed, led to widespread negligence of 'difficult' relatives or neighbours.[5] Scull went on to claim that the asylum was used to mould social 'misfits' towards acceptable middle-class cultural norms and expectations; any patients who were unable to conform remained incarcerated and subsequently silted up the asylum system. Scull accused the new mad-doctors of monopolizing the management of the insane for their own professional advancement, and attributed asylum growth (and their rising populations) to class interest.[6] Scull's work has been challenged; he pointed to how 'micro researches' often failed to engage with broader issues and were a rupture from wider historical contexts.[7] His claim that asylum histories had become too isolated and specific underestimates their contribution to the understanding of nineteenth-century psychiatric practices; they highlight the disparities and nuances which, although often localized, compel evidential reconsideration. Recently, historians have redressed the balance with studies grounded in detailed archival research rather than broad theory. Increasingly, asylum patients have been contextualized in carefully detailed and nuanced studies of individual institutions, and in the process the chronology of confinement and asylum growth has been challenged.[8] As Len Smith has explained, a 'mixed economy of care' survived the watershed legislation reforming asylums in 1845.[9] Work by Peter Bartlett has highlighted how Poor Law workhouses continued to provide care for the pauper insane long after that date, but rather less is known about continuities and differences following the 1845 legislation which began in a phase of therapeutic optimism that assumed (mistakenly) that most patients would be admitted at an early, and thus curable, stage of their illness.[10] *Institutionalizing the Insane* addresses this shortfall. By examining connections and differences, it shows that the realities of asylum care had an impact on medical confidence.

Issues of gender and class have featured in general histories of psychiatry and specific institutional studies; for example, Anne Digby's influential work on the Quaker-run York Retreat documented patients' different social backgrounds and treatment, as did Charlotte MacKenzie's comprehensive account of the private Ticehurst.[11] The rigid class distinctions of most aspects of Victorian life informed the belief that the segregation of pauper lunatics from the middle-class insane was appropriate and medically beneficial. This does not necessarily mean that Scull's view of institutional care of the insane being based on a class-based model reflective of societal structure and values is wholly correct.[12] Lorraine Walsh, for example, points out that this perception overlooks other contributory factors. She contends that 'respectability' associated with morality and independence was the concept valued and revered by the middle classes who managed the asylums.[13] 'Respectability' thus negates the relevance of assuming all pauper patients were poor and all private patients were rich. This holds true, not only for Brookwood and Holloway, but also for many other institutions, such as the Devon County Asylum or Denbigh Asylum.[14] As Walsh stated, it is overly simplistic to label such patients as merely 'pauper' or 'private', as this overlooks the influence of contemporary class perceptions on policy and asylum management.[15]

Just as class is problematic when it comes to understanding asylums, so too is gender. Women as psychiatric patients have exercised an enduring fascination for historians, with early studies focusing on them as primarily victims of misogynistic psychiatric practice, which ranged from the patronizing to the cruel and abusive.[16] Elaine Showalter and Jane Ussher presented women's incarceration as an extreme manifestation of a male bourgeois enforcement of the domestication of the weaker sex.[17] They provoked heated debate amongst social and medical historians and are still cited today, if only in refutation and as a starting point for more balanced perspectives on gender differences. However, in trying not to construct a 'hysterical' view of the nineteenth-century female patient, the rigidity and restrictiveness of women's lives and the way that this informed their incarceration and treatment in asylums, should not be underplayed.[18] The research on Brookwood Asylum and Holloway Sanatorium in this book considers both female and male patients so as to present a more nuanced view of the patient experience. That said, some aspects of female incarceration, as well as societal (and medical) expectations, remain unique.

Increasingly, the relevance of family and community relationships with the incarceration process has been recognized, as arguably first highlighted in John Walton's work on Lancaster Asylum. His 'casting out' and 'bringing back' of insane relatives was explored and family breakdown cited as one of the key factors within the committal process. He challenged the view of the nineteenth-century asylum as a 'dumping ground' for the indolent and unwanted members of an industrial society.[19] David Wright's work on the Buckinghamshire County Asylum at Stone emphasized the collaborative role of relatives. Rather than suggesting that the deterioration of the family as a cohesive unit was the trigger for resorting to asylum care, he proposed that relatives chose to place unmanageable family members under professional care and control. Wright's work on the family's involvement in the discharge process, in particular, led him to suggest that the confinement of the insane can be viewed as the household's considered and rational response to the pressures of industrialization and social change. *Institutionalizing the Insane* to some extent endorses this view, but explores the similarities and differences between the families' rationale for taking such action. The alleged stigma of certification for the middle classes is somewhat at odds with the fact that, as the nineteenth century progressed, increased numbers of the 'respectable' middle classes were to be found within the asylums.[20] This further suggests that the asylum was not necessarily considered by families as a last resort, and that attitudes towards institutional care were shifting. However, the stigma attached to the asylums never entirely disappeared, hence the usage of 'Sanatorium' for the Holloway institution.

Direct comparisons of asylum regimes are rare. One of the earliest is Elaine Dwyer's study of the development of two nineteenth-century state institutions in New York, USA, which contrasted the differences between the asylums and their patients. Both these institutions, however, catered for the pauper class, shared administrative and medical concerns but had different therapeutic goals; Utica (opened in 1843) was intended for the acute cases and Willard (1869) for the care of the chronically insane.[21] Latterly, the work of Melling and Forsythe surveyed the different types of institutional care available for Devon's insane and made an important contribution to the historiography, although they highlighted that the geographical area examined may not have been typical of other parts of England and that more research was required.[22] Their excellent and detailed quantitative analysis to some extent makes it more difficult to access the actuality of the asylum patient experience. *Institutionalizing the*

Insane offers a direct comparison of the key components of asylum life whilst including a considerable amount of personal material and case reconstructions that add an important human dimension to the analysis and, ultimately, to our understanding. Two distinct social groups of patients are compared; their characteristics, their admission patterns, illnesses and daily care. Treatments and the therapeutic environments are contrasted whilst taking into account the impact of class assumptions and gender differences on medical outcomes. The influence of the asylum doctors on the daily routine and general character of each asylum is also considered. Ultimately, their success was dependent on efficient and well-managed staff, and the duties and behaviour of the asylum attendants are examined in detail. Often staff moved between the two institutions for professional advancement, adding an interesting dimension to the analysis.

The stimulus for *Institutionalizing the Insane* is to challenge assumptions of the nineteenth-century asylum and of the institutional care offered to the insane. Some stereotyping and beliefs have persisted, such as the image of the county asylum as a 'warehouse' with no curative agenda; the preponderance of female patients, admitted in excessive numbers compared to their male counterparts; the collusion of male relatives with medical authorities in assigning awkward women to a life of incarceration; or the lack of interest or powerlessness of the pauper class in respect of their relatives' treatment. Employing a comparative approach that is grounded in extensive archival sources, the book endorses some earlier research on asylums, but reveals a far more nuanced picture of the complexities of nineteenth-century custodial care for the insane than has hitherto been drawn. Did Holloway and Brookwood have the same numbers of female patients? Were the same age groups represented? What were the long-term prospects for inmates, and is there evidence of discriminatory practices outside the sexual and cultural norms of the time? The patients at both asylums had the same illnesses, but the proportion and range of physical and medical therapies varied. Given that one was a public institution, and the other private, was it likely that there would be differences in treatment and outcomes?

By comparing two institutions intended for two distinct social groups, namely paupers and the middle classes, it is apparent that class was even more important than gender in determining patients' diagnosis, incarceration, treatment and outcomes. Gender does not 'disappear' as an analytic category, but it is less important here than might have been expected. The class-specific intentions of the two asylums are broadly confirmed, but there are interesting variables that corroborate some findings from other individual asylums. Given its size, did Brookwood primarily function as a 'warehouse' for the insane or did it provide a more benign environment for its patients and even attempt to operate as a place of scientific enquiry? Unimpeded by accountability to the ratepayers (although, of course, it was answerable to other bodies), it might be supposed that Holloway offered a substantially better package of care and treatment, and that as a result patients were safer and would recover and subsequently be discharged more quickly than their lower-class contemporaries. Was this in fact the reality? How impermeable were the asylums? The evidence here challenges earlier suggestions that they maintained an isolated and self-contained presence, by uncovering a more fluid relationship between the asylum and society.[23]

While documentary sources have formed the basis of the research, in order to effectively contrast these two institutions and the type of care that they offered, it was necessary to use some quantitative data to complement and substantiate the qualitative analysis. This was then built up and interpretations created from this substantive evidence.[24] The scale of enterprise was substantial, owing to the quantity of surviving material. The completeness of the Brookwood archives, in particular, has enabled fresh insights into life in a large nineteenth-century institution which remained important to the local community even after its closure in 1994. The official administrative records consulted were principally the Minutes of the Committee of Visitors and the House Committee as well as the detailed annual reports, and staff registers which provided some fascinating biographical snapshots of nineteenth-century attendants; these were further enhanced by a later discovery of additional letters and papers.

Whilst the majority of the Brookwood archives survived, those for Holloway Sanatorium are much less complete, primarily as a result of the hospital's closure in 1981 when much was lost or destroyed. The dispersal of Holloway's archives is regrettable. Despite this, it was possible to engage with a wide range of sources that provided extensive and comparable information on patients, staff, therapeutics and the asylum building which made a multifaceted, comparative study feasible.[25] Holloway's admissions provided invaluable data comparable to Brookwood, with additional demographic and personal details on the patients, including their medical condition. Holloway Sanatorium opened in 1885 and annual data was collected from opening to 1905. This allowed for sufficient information to manipulate and test hypotheses. As with Brookwood, the Holloway case books were invaluable in extracting more in-depth information and reconstruct cases studies.

Institutionalizing the Insane incorporates examples of private correspondence that shows often high levels of family involvement and collaboration in the incarceration and discharge of their relatives.[26] Evidence from letters written to and by the patients offers a rare opportunity to hear their perspectives, to assess family levels of involvement in their care, and to better understand the context and reality of the asylum experience. The scarcity of personal records has meant that the voices of the poor have not often been heard. Predictably, most surviving correspondence has originated from the more literate middle and upper classes, so the surviving Brookwood letters and notes are particularly unusual. Often surprisingly well-written, they demonstrate the trauma of separation.

Authors express anxiety about relatives' health, and many attempt to understand the processes involved in the detention of their loved ones. Holloway families and friends also involved themselves in the patients' post-admission care, as did the upper-class families of the Ticehurst patients.[27] This is perhaps unsurprising given their class and levels of literacy, and that many were paying for treatment. Less correspondence has survived from the Holloway families, who could stay at the sanatorium while relatives were undergoing treatment, which was an option not available at Brookwood. As Louise Wanell highlighted in her work on letters associated with the York retreat, such sources offer important insights into the 'human and emotional side' of the relationships between families and asylum doctors which cannot be gleaned from more official sources.[28]

Institutionalizing the Insane sets the context by providing a detailed introduction to Brookwood Asylum and Holloway Sanatorium. The class-orientated rationale that informed their design, construction and governance are examined closely and an introduction to the general patient populations is followed by a specific comparison of the admissions to Brookwood and Holloway.[29] The superintendent and his staff were crucial for the stability and success of any asylum, and Chapter 2 examines the importance of the first superintendents, Dr Brushfield at Brookwood and Dr Rees Philipps at Holloway, as well as their long careers and influence in the profession. Their roles were complex and demanding; rapid growth made delegation essential as the superintendents struggled to keep abreast of ever-increasing medical and administrative demands. Until the end of the nineteenth century, asylum doctors were 'almost exclusively' male and, reflective of society, women tended to assume subordinate roles in the asylum hierarchy, such as nurse, housekeeper or, at best, matron.[30] This was the case at Brookwood, and initially at Holloway, but unusually, by the late 1890s, the sanatorium employed a succession of female medical officers who were highly valued by the superintendent.

Doctors and senior medical staff acted as agents of care; their decisions decided the therapeutic regime and any successful implementation depended on the attendants' efficiency, particularly with regard to suicidal patients.[31] Increasingly, the importance of the attendants in all aspects of treatment and care was recognized.[32] Living in such close proximity to the patients, asylum staff exerted an important moral influence and so the attendants were subjected to close observation and strict rules. This chapter looks at the difficulties of engaging and retaining competent, compassionate staff and the personal and professional qualities that were required. Many female attendants left their jobs to marry, but a significant number of married couples were employed to the advantage of both asylums. What methods were used to address class-specific issues of patient care? At Holloway, the superintendent engaged a small number of educated and genteel carers to live among the upper and middle class patients, acting as companions.

Chapter 3 looks at the patients in more detail, measuring and comparing admissions, discharges, ages and classifications of illness for both asylums. The gender representation is examined and the impact of the large numbers of chronic patients on asylum life is considered. Most Brookwood patients, particularly the younger men, were transferred directly from the workhouses. Patient admissions were not entirely in the hands of the medical profession, but also depended on the families' desire for effective and safe custodial care for difficult and often violent relatives. Wright concluded that the confinement of the insane was often a 'pragmatic response of households to the stresses of industrialization', as opposed to the desire of a medical elite seeking professionalization.[33] Families' influence intersected with that of the medical authorities in their accounts of the patients' behaviour, as well as in the collaboration on treatment and the period of institutional care. The letters and case books provide insights into the relationship between patients' families and medical authorities, illustrating the extent of family influence on incarceration and discharge which is contrasted between the two asylums. No patients under the age of fifteen years were admitted to Holloway, but Brookwood cared for several small children, many of whom are described as 'imbeciles' or 'idiots'. They came either from workhouses, or were brought in by desperate parents seeking respite, although some later regretted this and tried to reclaim them.[34] Although they represented a small patient subgroup at Brookwood, they were of great managerial concern. Children in nineteenth-century asylums have been largely ignored hitherto, and this study begins to address this neglect.

Chapter 4 examines the residential patients of the two asylums in more detail and new perspectives are offered on sex ratios, age and marital status. Patient occupations reveal a less homogenous class-based patient population than might have been predicted. Some patients could be defined as middle class, or as skilled working class, and would not have been classified officially as paupers. So why did their relatives chose the pauper asylum? The associated costs for mental health care were prohibitive for many, and it can be surmised that many families were unable or unwilling to afford the expense. Personal correspondence indicates a wide range of circumstances and reasons for the incarceration of relatives in the respective asylums.

The research presented here refutes earlier claims by Scull that a silted-up county asylum system merely warehoused the old, infirm and unwanted members of society and that private asylums were 'institutions for private imprisonment' and just as unlikely to be able to cure their patients. The evidence from Brookwood and Holloway endorses the work of Laurence Ray and David Wright, who concluded that the long-term confinement of patients was in fact, exceptional.[35] MacKenzie has pointed out that the discharge rates at Ticehurst were similar to those of public institutions with little evidence of patients being incarcerated for years on end. Further, accusations of social control are less appropriate in the private sector than within the public sector, where there was a class difference between the incarcerated and their keepers.[36] Such class issues at Holloway were partially addressed by the engagement of middle-class 'companions' as well as by the superintendent incorporating his interpretation of middle-class propriety into his management strategy. Class definitions within the asylum were problematic at Holloway; only patients who met the Board's 'criteria' were considered suitable for admission and/or worthy of charitable assistance.[37]

Female patients at both institutions were subjected to distinctive contemporary cultural expectations; medical 'experts' of the day have referred to female frailty and their propensity for mental instability, but there is little gender disparity within the asylum admissions. However, the evidence from Brookwood and Holloway reveals that the important factor is the over-representation of women in the *residual* asylum populations; they accounted for most of the 'chronic' patients, and formed the bulk of the voluntary boarders staying indefinitely at Holloway. This chapter offers some explanations for this. Madness was often seen to manifest itself in inappropriate female behaviour, such as bad language, lack of interest in their children or household matters, and overt sexual conduct. Some historians have examined how the diagnosis and treatment of peculiarly female mental disorders, such as hysteria and depression, were allegedly used to 'entrap' women in their biological destiny.[38] This association is particularly relevant for women who suffered from puerperal insanity, or who committed infanticide, and the prescribed treatments were influenced by the strength of belief in the woman's natural role in society.[39] The first medical superintendents at both institutions believed that women were more prone to mental disorder which was usually less severe than that endured by men. As a result, their recovery was quicker, and in addition they apparently benefited from being immune to certain conditions such as GPI or serious suicidal ideation. As gender studies evolved to consider perceptions of male identity, so have certain mental illnesses ascribed to men come to the fore, for example shell-shock. That said, the focus on gender-specific diagnosis remains primarily on women. The often self-destructive relationship between women and food appears more frequently in the Holloway records; anorexia nervosa was seen as symptomatic of melancholia and so sufferers were perceived as a suicide risk. Although some men also refused food, the records show that this behaviour was more common in women.[40]

The return to socially acceptable behaviour was viewed as a prime indicator of recovery for women in particular. Patient cure and the restoration of 'normal' behaviour are dealt with in Chapter 5. Treatment was prescribed after the initial examination and diagnosis given on admission, the accuracy of which was often hindered by a lack of information that accompanied the new patient. Perceptions of the patient's social standing also significantly shaped doctors' opinions and any prescribed therapeutics. Regardless of the patients' class, most treatment was based on moral therapy, occasionally supplemented by physical activity and limited chemical treatments. Poor general health undermined the efficacy of what, admittedly, were the limited options available at Brookwood, but this may not have resulted in the asylum having less success than Holloway.

Moral treatment essentially rejected physical restraint but required patient co-operation. It encompassed the entire asylum environment and regime, with every detail and component of daily life seen as contributing to therapeutic success. Despite the volume of patients and limited resources, Brookwood's management largely resisted the pessimism of some late Victorian asylum regimes and were actually successful in implementing regulated and gender-segregated work programmes. The majority of patients participated and only the elderly or the ill were exempt. The work-centred approach was initially less effective at Holloway, as manual labour was an alien concept for many patients, but this did gradually alter over the years. At Holloway, there was always a stronger emphasis on recreation as a therapeutic device and an extensive range of amusements was available to all Holloway patients. Brookwood also provided amusements, but these were fewer, less extravagant and more likely to be restricted to within the asylum.[41] At Holloway innovative treatments included massage, electricity and shower baths and they used a wider range of chemical therapies on a regular basis than at Brookwood.

The existence of suicidal tendencies amongst some asylum patients was one specific aspect of mental illness that caused a great deal of medical and lay consternation. Self-destructive behaviour was often the catalyst for families to seek professional help for their relatives.[42] Chapter 6 addresses the asylum's response to suicidal behaviour and questions the incidence of suicidal patients. How did Brookwood Asylum and Holloway Sanatorium manage and protect these vulnerable patients and how successful were they? The Holloway management, ever mindful of middle-class propriety, employed minimally intrusive strategies, so that there were several completed suicides within the sanatorium. The stricter practices put into place by the (much larger) public asylum of Brookwood were ultimately more effective in suicide prevention. Illustrated by examples from the case books and letters from both institutions, this chapter shows yet another dimension in this multifaceted comparative asylum study.

By the early nineteenth century, there was a perceptible shift from suicide being a predominantly religious and legal concern, to one in which the medical profession had a dominant role. Olive Anderson showed that this reconfiguration of suicide as symptomatic of mental illness was beneficial to many agencies.[43] Asylum superintendents pressed the case for institutional care and control. They asserted that self-destruction could be prevented if there was professional intervention early enough in the illness. Anderson's work reinforced the impression, given by the Lunacy Commissioners in 1882, that the asylum was an effective force in the prevention of suicide and the supervision of the suicidal.[44] More recent work has built upon this, considering the realities of caring for these patients and the importance of the asylum and the attendants in suicide prevention.[45]

There have been challenges in reconstructing the parallel histories of these two institutions, including the volume and range of sources, missing material and the uneven recording mechanisms within the institutions themselves. However, the end result demonstrates that it is both possible, and valuable, to contrast mental health care provision in two distinct sets of nineteenth-century patients. While it has not been possible to be all-inclusive, this book highlights and examines the main protagonists in the unfolding narrative of psychiatric care at this time; the buildings that provided the therapeutic environment, the doctors and attendants who supervised and provided the medical care, the patients as recipients of this care, and the nature of the therapy and the likelihood of recovery. Suicidal behaviour, or rather its control, was considered as an indicator of therapeutic success. Cultural assumptions regarding gender and class influenced the diagnosis, treatment and outcomes for patients, but the authorities did not act alone, and this book clearly highlights the importance of family interaction and expectations.

The challenges and limitations of working with patient case notes have been well documented; one of the principle drawbacks is that they can only ever provide the medical perspective and thus contain inherent class and professional prejudices. However, they are invaluable in helping to decipher social attitudes towards the insane. When combined with other official asylum records (annual reports, dispensary and financial records etc.) they offer important information on asylum diagnostics, therapeutics and regimes. Where they are arguably less helpful, is in providing evidence from the patient's perspective, or that of their families. For this reason, selected letters from families and patients are used here, in order to facilitate understanding of the patient experience, and the impact of poverty on mental illness in nineteenth-century Surrey. They offer an important avenue of investigation as they allow an attempted reconstruction of the patient experience integrated with historical analyses.[46] Their value is enhanced by the fact that most were written during the illness, not after recovery, and so are not affected by hindsight and reflection. There has been no previous comparison of the role of middle-class patients and their families with that of poor or pauper patients and families. *Institutionalizing the Insane* begins to address this while acknowledging that it can only be one, albeit important, aspect.[47]

At Brookwood the evidence challenges the notion of powerless and inarticulate pauper families and, at Holloway, questions the motives of the middle-class families who wished to have their relatives cared for in luxurious circumstance. By comparing and contrasting these two Surrey institutions and by investigating the strength of their common approach to key therapies, the persistent images of the pauper and private asylum regimes are challenged, and new insights offered into the lives of their patients and staff. These insights are amplified by hearing the voices of those families in receipt of mental health care in the nineteenth century.

1 CARING FOR SURREY'S INSANE: BROOKWOOD ASYLUM AND HOLLOWAY SANATORIUM

Introduction

Nineteenth-century Surrey encompassed both crowded urban settlements in south London and a sprawling rural population. As the county's population increased, so too did the numbers of lunatics requiring care and control. The first Surrey County Asylum, Springfield, opened at Wandsworth in 1841 with 299 patients and was soon filled beyond capacity.[1] This necessitated the creation of Brookwood, a second asylum at Woking, which was opened on 17 June 1867 by the Metropolitan Asylums Board (MAB), the new authority created to care for the infectious and insane poor of Greater London.[2] In contrast, the nearby Holloway Sanatorium was established by private bequest for the exclusive benefit of the middle-class insane. It relied on the fees of the better-off patients to subsidize those less affluent but who were deemed as 'deserving' of assistance. Philanthropic support to create and support hospitals increased as the nineteenth century progressed.[3] Holloway was completed in 1884, being described as 'the most grandiloquent of all nineteenth-century donations' both in the size and scale of the building and in its lavish interior.[4]

This chapter compares and contrasts the two very different psychiatric institutions, considering the admissions and management structure, and daily routines. As suggested earlier, asylums have been associated with increased professionalization, unfair and lengthy confinement and social control. Pauper institutions in particular, were often defined as warehouses for societal misfits whose problems were medicalized.[5] The smaller private asylums, with fewer patients and financial constraints, ostensibly offered a better standard of care, but, as shall be seen, this did not necessarily offer greater safety for the patients.

Origins

Brookwood Asylum

When Springfield opened in 1841, Surrey's general population was already upwards of 557,000 and reached 718,549 in 1901.[6] Initially, most of Brookwood's patients originated from the urban parts of the county, which included deprived, populous areas in south London such as Rotherhithe, Bermondsey and Southwark.[7] Bermondsey was home to some noxious industries, including a substantial leather works and glue factory, as well as food processing and canning plants. Nearby, the Rotherhithe docks had been a major whaling base until the 1840s, after which they were replaced by timber yards. Many factories were built in the Southwark area as the river facilitated the transport of raw materials and finished goods. These industries, concentrated within a relatively small area, brought with them all the social problems associated with rapid migration. Overcrowding, poor quality housing, poverty, crime and deprivation were its defining characteristics.[8] Nearby Camberwell, however, was slightly more affluent, as it was primarily a mixed residential area with no industry.[9] Neighbouring Wandsworth was a thriving and busy district that boasted many fine houses but, unlike Camberwell, it was also a commercial centre with oil mills, dye works, paper and corn mills, calico printing works, vinegar works, distilleries and a thriving brewery. Some of these trades were represented amongst Brookwood's inmates, but so, too, was evidence of the unemployment that plagued casual labourers and employees.

Even before Brookwood was officially opened, the management was besieged by requests to accommodate pauper lunatics from workhouses in deprived areas of south London. They resisted numerous requests to admit many aged, infirm and other 'undesirables', for fear of opening the floodgates to incurable or inappropriate patients. However, it was impossible to exclude all such cases, and the records frequently describe ex-workhouse patients who arrived in very poor physical and mental condition. The sheer volume of all admissions stretched administrative and medical resources to the utmost, and a third Surrey public asylum was eventually opened at Cane Hill in 1884. In addition, private institutions, both inside and outside the county, were used to accommodate pauper lunatics until spaces became available within the rate-aided institutions.

As early as 1836, rural Surrey was identified as a prime location for a public asylum; land was reasonably priced and an abundance of open countryside made it feasible to purchase a large plot which would not curtail any necessary future building work, should it be required.[10] By 1854, Springfield was obliged to turn away patients who then had to be accommodated elsewhere until beds became free. The management discussed expanding the asylum but by 1860, this idea was discarded due to the cost.[11] Instead, a site for a new asylum was sought, and eventually:

The Committee, after a laborious search and prolonged inquiry, selected a locality possessing in a remarkable degree, the principal requirements, a healthy aspect, a fine free air, and being a spot easily approached from various points of the County by convergence at Woking of several railroads traversing the district.[12]

Plans for a new institution elicited mixed responses from the local boards of guardians. In 1859, the rural Chertsey Union had reported the inadequacies of the urban Springfield asylum and recommended that 'if any increased accommodation is absolutely required, it should be obtained by the erection of an Asylum in the more rural parts of the County, on the most economical plan'. The priorities were: 'abundant open space, land of low value, and the most favourable climate'.[13] Initially, magistrates (who still played a significant role in the administration of the insane) resisted the idea of a new, more rurally based asylum, arguing that patients benefited from localized accommodation close to their relatives in order to achieve swifter rehabilitation.[14] Early resistance from local boards of guardians arose partially from financial concerns as workhouse maintenance costs were lower than those of a county asylum.[15] The Guildford Board of Guardians also emphasized its belief that certain lunatics, chiefly imbeciles and chronic cases, benefited from being cared for in the workhouses as they were fed a superior diet and remained in close proximity to their families and communities.[16] Brookwood's newly elected Committee of Visitors did acknowledge that workhouses might have some part to play in the accommodation of lunatics but stipulated that this was strictly *in the short term*.[17]

Cheap land and good rail communications made rural Surrey generally attractive for building large institutions, including Brookwood, and offered the potential to absorb the 'problem populations' from the rapidly expanding capital. The land, a 150-acre plot with scenic views, was bought from the London Necropolis and National Mausoleum Company for £10,500.[18] At the 1862 Epiphany Quarter Sessions, the Committee of Visitors was instructed to approach the Commissioners in Lunacy to appoint 'some competent architect'. Charles Henry Howell was chosen; he was Surrey's County Surveyor from 1860, and also architect to the Commissioners in Lunacy.[19] As advised, Howell visited several asylums in England and France for inspiration.[20] Keenly aware of problems that Wandsworth's spatial limitations had caused Surrey's lunatic poor, the committee was anxious to oversee the construction of a cost-effective institution that would obviate the necessity for immediate expansion. The intention was for the asylum to be largely self-sufficient, with the capacity to establish a farm where patients would grow their own food. This also provided necessary employment for refractory patients, and thus conformed to contemporary notions of moral treatment, as did the asylum's relative isolation.[21]

Holloway Sanatorium

For many of the emergent middle classes, Poor Law institutions embodied the stigma of family mental disorder, but private or fee-paying establishments were often beyond their means. Despite some adverse publicity, the demand for private care continued as families increasingly sought treatment for afflicted relatives.[22] This requirement corresponded with a growing medical interest in the links between insanity and hereditary disorder. The middle and upper classes favoured registered hospitals and, to a much lesser degree, private accommodation in public asylums rather than licensed houses. But any form of private care was costly for middle-class families; as early as 1750, the Trustees for St Luke's Hospital for Lunatics, London, declared that the rationale for their new establishment was, 'that the expense necessarily attending the confinement and other means of cure are such as people born in middling circumstances cannot bear'.[23] Thomas Holloway created the Holloway Sanatorium at Virginia Water specifically to benefit the middle-class insane; this was a response to the perceived financial vulnerability of the middle class and because patients from this class were considered to have been largely excluded from appropriate, and affordable, institutional psychiatric care. Once open, Holloway's management continually compared and measured their success against the performance of other establishments, including St Luke's. Keen to emphasize that it considered itself as a hospital, and not an asylum, St Luke's operated a system of 'disqualifying rules'.[24] A century later, Holloway Sanatorium followed suit, striving to ensure that it did not become a moribund custodial institution. It also admitted some subsidized patients as a charitable endeavour, as did the York Retreat.[25]

The issue of where to send the middle-class insane was much debated during the mid-nineteenth century. An 1859 Parliamentary Select Committee included Lord Shaftesbury (first chairman of the Commissioners in Lunacy) as the chief witness.[26] It concluded that it was inappropriate for the middle classes to be incarcerated with the pauper class for any length of time, and that it was even detrimental to patient recovery. Shaftesbury considered that:

> Asylums where there are not a number of proprietors looking for profit present the very greatest advantages; and I find that patients are taken into them at a lower figure than at any private house, and the richer patients who go into these asylums, by the larger sum they pay, contribute from the overplus to alleviate the burdens upon the poorer inmates.[27]

At a public meeting held two years after the Select Committee, Shaftesbury tried to raise funds for an asylum specifically for this class of patient, but with little success.[28] Thomas Holloway attended this meeting and was inspired by Shaftesbury's commitment. They began to meet privately, and Holloway started to plan the fulfilment of Shaftesbury's vision.[29]

Thomas Holloway (1800–83) was a wealthy patent medicine manufacturer and philanthropist. His business thrived through extensive advertising of his pills and ointments. By the 1870s, he was reputedly making more than £50,000 a year in profit.[30] Married but childless, and with a considerable personal fortune, Holloway sought outlets for his money that would also constitute a permanent testimonial to his spectacular rise from humble origins. He decided upon two major projects: Holloway Sanatorium for the insane middle classes, and the nearby Royal Holloway College for the education of women.

Thomas Holloway stated that 'Charity demeans the recipient of charity'.[31] This view was broadly in keeping with contemporary political economists, who perceived charity as creating a culture of dependence. They advocated a more rational and scientific approach to philanthropy. Certainly, Holloway's philanthropic principle, broadly speaking, was that help should only be given to the deserving. By his definition, this meant those who had previously exhibited the work ethic, and had abandoned it only because of necessity or ill fortune. Something of an enigma, with few surviving clues as to his personality, the personal motivation that lay behind two mammoth projects of this pronounced recluse is not entirely clear. It has been suggested that Holloway possessed a 'London shopkeeper mentality' allied to liberal radicalism that prompted him to offer opportunities for the lower middle classes. He was certainly closely associated with some London radical reformers who also assisted him with these two ambitious projects.[32]

Why did the sanatorium take so long to create? Although Holloway's quest to create a 'Model place' was an ongoing concern, his business affairs – and his new residence at Sunningdale (close to the site eventually chosen for the sanatorium) – took precedence.[33] Nevertheless, Holloway spent much time researching the feasibility of building an insane asylum for the middle classes that was within easy reach of London. He visited asylums both abroad and in Britain (possibly at Shaftesbury's recommendation), including Brentwood, Hayward's Heath, Hanwell and Bridgend; the last was presided over at that time by Dr David Yellowlees, whom Holloway greatly admired.[34]

Holloway corresponded with the Commissioners in Lunacy and with architects, including George Godwin.[35] In early 1871, Holloway enlisted Godwin's help, and in a series of anonymous articles headed 'How to Spend Money for the Public Good' he solicited public opinion regarding his plans for a charitable establishment, and announced his proposed investment of some £300,000.[36] Suggestions were submitted, but the *Builder* declared that 'the great majority [were] utterly worthless'.[37] Despite Godwin's advice to appoint a selection panel, Thomas purchased a 22-acre site from Corpus Christi College, Oxford at St Ann's Heath, Virginia Water on his own initiative. It was here that he proposed building the first, in what he hoped would be a series, of hospitals for the afflicted middle-class insane.

In 1872 Holloway and Godwin organized a competition to choose the architect.[38] The entrants were provided with sixteen pages of guidance that followed prescripts of traditional asylum layout and general requirements. Holloway was, however, very specific on detail and he was able to provide instructions as to where particular products could be viewed *in situ* or where the manufacturers could be found.[39] He wanted his asylum to possess innovative facilities and to be 'a model institution' that was 'free from "ruts"'.[40]

The selection panel included asylum legislation experts, as well as medical practitioners such as Dr Yellowlees and Dr Lockhart Robertson (of Hayward's Heath Asylum), as well as the architect Thomas Henry Wyatt, who was co-designer of the county asylums for Wiltshire and Buckinghamshire. From thirteen designs, the panel finally chose 'Alpha' by William Henry Crossland (1834–1908).[41] Despite having chosen the competition winner, the panel cautioned that 'there is not one of the designs which would not require more or less modification of plan and general arrangement ere it could be carried into execution for practical working'.[42] Holloway's desire to build an institution that would be a worthy and fitting testimony to his munificence was tempered by his thrifty disposition. This prompted modifications such as using Portland Stone dressings (Holloway's choice) over ornamental brick (preferred by Crossland). This and many other alterations to the original plan resulted in a diminution of Flemish style and less 'pure' Gothic. It is fairly certain that the building which eventually opened in 1885 was vastly different from the competition plan submitted in 1872, which unfortunately has not survived.[43]

The concern to provide a luxurious environment with the most up-to-date equipment overrode more practical considerations of providing secure and legally compliant accommodation for patients. *Building News*, whilst paying tribute to the competition entrants, baldly stated that their evident talent and style did not necessarily mean they were capable of designing an asylum.[44] Furthermore, the journal opined that the Commissioners in Lunacy would be unlikely to pass any of the competition plans in their existing format.[45] From the onset Holloway must have been aware of potential pitfalls and of the necessity of complying with lunacy legislation, yet these early warnings regarding the unsuitability of the accommodation went largely unheeded and the building possessed serious shortcomings that delayed the opening and plagued its early years.

The first brick was laid by Jane Holloway (Thomas's wife) in spring 1873 and the main contractors began work that summer. Initial progress was fairly rapid, and in 1877 the *Builder* claimed that the sanatorium was 'approaching completion', as the main building was already roofed in.[46] The interior designing had been commissioned, including the richly decorated halls, entrance and staircase. By 1878, the sanatorium was virtually finished, yet it was another seven years before it opened to receive patients. One possible reason for the delay may have been that the College project had become more of a priority for Holloway.[47] The death of Holloway's wife Jane in 1875 and his own illness from 1877 were further likely factors. By 1884, the substantial delay combined with additional work that included building the chapel, landscaping and planting the grounds, had caused costs to escalate to over £300,000. When it finally opened, the sanatorium had cost over five times the cost per patient of a publicly funded asylum built to the standards of the Commissioners in Lunacy.[48]

Only 20 miles from London, and conveniently accessible by rail, the sanatorium attested to the importance of the metropolis as a source of potential patients. For years before it opened, there had been considerable public interest in both the outstanding architecture as well as in the intended clientele. While building was in progress, Thomas Holloway utilized the site's closeness to the South-Western Railway by erecting a huge sign facing the railway bridge that for nine years proclaimed the forthcoming opening of Holloway Sanatorium for the care of mental diseases in persons of the middle class.[49]

Thomas Holloway never saw the completion of his ambitious project; he died of lung congestion in December 1883. Within the year, the sanatorium was furnished, fully equipped, insured, and Dr Sutherland Rees Philipps was appointed as the first medical superintendent.[50] The management of Holloway Sanatorium was taken on by Holloway's two brothers-in-law, Henry Driver Holloway and George Martin Holloway, who strove to enshrine the founder's ideals in the daily running of the hospital, which finally opened to receive patients in June 1885.[51]

Buildings and Environment

Brookwood Asylum

The 1808 Asylums Act (or Wynn's Act) empowered local magistrates to build rate-aided institutions to care for their insane poor and also provided guidance for their construction and management. As Len Smith has pointed out, despite its limitations, the Act provided the strategic basis for the English asylum system.[52] Local authorities progressed slowly but steadily in this field, although this occurred mainly in the provinces. The particular issue of London's pauper lunacy went largely unaddressed until a Select Committee in 1827 prompted plans to construct the Middlesex County Asylum at Hanwell, which opened in 1830.[53] In 1845, further legislation made borough and county provision compulsory and installed a national inspectorate which was responsible for both public and private asylums.[54]

Local justices sought prime sites in an 'airy and healthy' situation, often on the outskirts of a town or city, although this had not always been the case. Asylums built in the late eighteenth and early nineteenth century had often been built in urban areas, for example, Bethlem and St Luke's. The medical profession expressed some concern that their location undermined efforts to impose moral treatment, which was strongly refuted by their respective superintendents.[55] Finding a suitable remote, yet accessible site reflected medical concerns about the necessity of separating the insane from their usual surroundings. Given that urban dwelling was, for many, associated with moral deprivation and inequity, the asylum and its inhabitants should benefit from a natural, tranquil and rural setting.[56]

In 1854, John Conolly had highlighted the particular desirability of the Surrey countryside as being ideal for an asylum.[57] Brookwood's site was only 3 miles from Woking and 1 mile from Brookwood railway station. As had been debated in the *Asylum Journal*, accessibility by rail was especially important, not only for easily transporting patients from the metropolis, but also to prevent the asylum from becoming isolated from resources, ideas and medical developments.[58] As will be shown, the relative isolation of both asylums was problematic for some members of staff and also for the patients, particularly so at Holloway.

Brookwood enjoyed extensive views of the surrounding countryside; its 150 acres sloped down to the south where it was bound by the Basingstoke Canal and on the east and west by the main roads to Guildford and Chertsey. Reporting on his visit to the proposed site with the architect, Charles Howell, Justice Robert Rawlinson extolled its advantages, including accessibility, the quality of the soil, the healthy climate and the sufficiency of water (although in common with many other asylums at the time, this was later found not to be the case).[59]

The asylum building itself had to be practical to ensure security and supervision, reflecting the twin objectives of cure and custody, in short 'combining elements of both the penitentiary and the infirmary'.[60] Brookwood Asylum was constructed in stock brickwork, relieved by a few coloured brick dressings.[61] The main body was built in the popular 'H' layout, with a three-storied block and retreating wings to accommodate the sick and the newly admitted cases prior to assessment and subsequent categorization. The main block contained offices and patients' dormitories and, nearby, additional two-storey blocks housed the laundry, workshops and further patient accommodation, primarily for 'working' and convalescing patients. Covered walkways connected all the main buildings.[62] The grounds were spacious enough to contain additional houses, such as the superintendent's, as well as cottages large enough for the gardener and the farm bailiff to be able to provide supervised accommodation for up to twelve 'quiet' patients each.[63] This arrangement allowed selected patients to form a semi-independent community under the supervision of the asylum regime; this emphasized Brookwood's therapeutic aspect and was unusual in pauper asylums at that time. A relatively plain chapel, for 343 people, was located within 200 yards of the main building. The architect was proud to report that all this had been achieved for the sum of £61,900.[64]

In his first annual report, the superintendent, Dr Brushfield, described Brookwood's accommodation as being bright and cheerful, with rooms that 'command good views of the surrounding country'.[65] There was no necessity for any frivolous or superfluous decoration, nor for any of the types of amenities that were soon to be provided for the middle-class insane at Holloway Sanatorium. Brookwood was essentially a utilitarian institution that provided adequate facilities in keeping with current ideas of lunacy provision and treatment. The lack of decorative excess was precisely in line with contemporary thinking on public asylum design, which favoured the plain and functional. Not only was this a responsible use of public funds, but better for the patient's well-being. As succinctly expressed by Dr Conolly in his *Lectures on the Construction and Government of Lunatic Asylums*: 'Much ornament or decoration, external or internal, is useless, and rather offends irritable patients than gives any satisfaction to the more contented'.[66]

The entire asylum environment contributed to the therapeutic effect, and the asylum grounds played an important part in providing opportunities for exercise and patient employment. Whether at private or public asylums, grounds were principally modelled on the aristocratic landscape park that combined an ornament with a functional, agricultural self-sufficiency. There were some necessary modifications, such as the addition of enclosed airing or exercise courts that would not be found at a stately home.[67] The airing courts, one each for men and women, were near the south side of the asylum and had sunken fences (similar to the main perimeter wall) to maintain the patients' uninterrupted rural view.[68] Brookwood's Head Gardener for some thirty years, Robert Lloyd (1833–1900), also designed the asylum grounds, and later worked closely with Howell, Brookwood's architect, on the grounds at Cane Hill Asylum as well as other asylum gardens.[69] Living at Brookwood, Lloyd and his wife also cared for patients in their cottage.[70]

The asylum interior conveyed the requisite utility and plainness, with the addition of the necessary practicalities, usually for safety, which reinforced its custodial function. The patients predominantly slept in dormitories; 594 initially, with a further 56 accommodated in single rooms that were fitted with locked shutters, doors which opened outwards flush to the wall and cast-iron door frames. Beds and furniture were plain, though 'of the best materials', usually birch. Windows had locks that allowed only a five-inch opening to limit opportunities for escape or suicide. With the addition of simple furniture, pictures and books, the aim was to create a homely and domestic environment, which for many patients would have been far superior to their usual living conditions.

There were problems. The asylum's heating did not work properly for years, with open fireplaces in the dormitories and dayrooms which were ineffectual in the corridors and single rooms which remained exceedingly cold; the infirmary was pronounced the coldest place of all.[71] Water supplies were erratic so that bathing and laundry were frequently suspended for short periods in summer – and the addition of a water tower and reservoirs holding over one million gallons of water seemingly did little to alleviate this problem.

Brookwood's management was soon obliged to address the rising numbers of applications for admission. Originally the asylum was intended for 650 inmates, but ambitious extension plans had to commence almost immediately and building work took place intermittently from 1874 to 1938. Major projects included new accommodation on both male and female sides which begun in 1875.[72] A self-contained cottage hospital was also built in the grounds, to act as an isolation facility for fever patients.[73] By 1938, Brookwood housed 1753 inmates.

Holloway Sanatorium

Holloway's concentration on beauty and luxury led to the oversight of some basic legal requirements. Problems surfaced as early as 1877 when the Commissioners in Lunacy refused the building a licence. Recent legislative changes required that all rooms occupied by patients had to open onto a corridor with a staircase that should lead directly outside in case of fire.[74] A chapel had not been included in the original plans but, as this was later stipulated by law, building commenced in 1882. Although Holloway was himself a Nonconformist, the sanatorium's chapel was resolutely Anglican in both character and ritual.[75]

Despite Holloway's impressive design and location, its first superintendent, Rees Philipps, was perturbed by its shortcomings. Upon his appointment, he observed that some 'prime requirements' were deficient:

> There were no corridors of communication in the portions of the building intended for occupation by the patients. The rooms opened into one another, so that there would have been no privacy for the patients, and great difficulty in administration. All meals for patients residing in the wings would have to be carried through several of the principal sitting rooms.[76]

Anticipating the type of patients that would stay at Holloway Sanatorium, expansive suites of rooms had been built across the front of the patient accommodation, with access via staircases at the rear for patients' own servants. Fire regulations were contravened, not least by the corridors' narrowness, which had been highlighted as early as 1872.[77] Charles Dorman, architect to St Andrew's Hospital Northampton, (a hospital admired by Rees Philipps) was quickly engaged, together with a local builder, to address the shortcomings. In addition to the corridors, extra storerooms and pantries connected to patient galleries were required, more staircases to act as fire escapes, as well as fewer partitions to allow more light into patient accommodation. Sanitary arrangements were overhauled by installing a new flush system, and the water supply was improved. New gas works were built in the grounds, electric light installed, the superintendent's accommodation extended and improved, and paths and roads laid out.

On the women's side a walled garden for the exercise of 'troublesome' female patients and two padded rooms were constructed.[78] Crossland's design was thereby brought up to date.

Just three days before the official opening, the Commissioners in Lunacy certified the sanatorium as suitable to receive 200 patients. The ceremony on 15 June 1885 was presided over by the Prince of Wales, who travelled with his retinue from nearby Ascot races. The occasion was reported by the local press, which praised the deceased Holloway and his charitable intention 'to provide a home for persons temporarily deprived of their reason, at charges suited to their means'.[79] The superior accommodation was much admired:

> For persons whose friends are opulent there are front rooms or suites of rooms and for others less fortunate apartments in less prominent parts of the building. But for all, rich or poor, is provided the same bright surroundings, and everything calculated to create an interest in those of our fellow creatures who are inmates of the Sanatorium.[80]

The hospital was designed in a popular layout of 'block and corridor'. A three-storey main building comprised a central portion that focused on a seven-bay high-roofed hall, flanked by subordinate sections of nineteen-bay apartment ranges on each side, one for female patients and one for males. An impressive terrace, 530 feet in length, ran across the front and a formidable central tower, 145 feet high, dominated the whole area. The chapel was built in French Gothic style.[81] Inside the sanatorium, there were spacious public rooms, including an 80 feet by 40 feet high-ceilinged recreation hall. This featured a 60-feet high hammer beam roof, elaborate gilding and portraits of distinguished figures, both contemporary and historical, including Thomas and Jane Holloway. There was a prominent featured statue of Thomas Holloway, as well as a 'striking portrait' and monograms of the Holloway initials and his adopted coat of arms, a decorative scheme that was particularly intense at the entrance to the reception hall.[82] Holloway thus ensured that patients and visitors to the sanatorium could not forget at whose behest the hospital had been built and would appreciate its superiority over other institutions. Contemporary commentary suggests that he more than achieved this. Compare the descriptions of Holloway with that of the much earlier St Luke's Hospital. The following was written shortly after St Luke's opened to receive charitable middle-class patients: 'a neat but very plain edifice; nothing here is expended in ornament and we only see a building of considerable length, plastered over and whitened, with ranges of small square windows on which no decorations have been bestowed'.[83]

Holloway's dining and recreation halls were designed and decorated to provide cheerfulness and distraction for troubled minds; 'cold and grey columns and walls, even if enlivened by sculpture would, it was considered, sit heavily on a mind diseased'.[84] The lavish interior had caused the *Builder* to exclaim: 'Such a combination of rich colouring and gilding is not to be found in any modern building in this country, except the House of Lords.'[85] Not everyone was quite so complimentary; after visiting Holloway Sanatorium in 1885, the young designer and architect Charles Ashbee observed that 'The decoration of the asylum is very garish and ghastly but appropriate'.[86]

Admissions and their Management

Following the 1845 legislation, a delicate balance between lay and professional concerns had been sought within asylum managerial practices; these were influenced by local factors, ambitious medical officers and committees of justices charged with protecting the interests of the patients and the public.[87] County justices, through Quarter Sessions, appointed a supervisory committee of visiting justices to oversee the asylums. From setting staff wages, paying for repairs, to ordering the discharge of cured patients, they possessed, as Smith has suggested, a considerable variety of discretionary powers.[88] As mentioned above, from 1845 both private and public institutions were overseen and inspected by a central body, the Commissioners in Lunacy.

Admissions to Brookwood

Reporting to the Quarter Sessions at Kingston, Brookwood's Committee of Visitors met on the third Friday of every month at 11.30 am to consider applications for admission. The management of these applications was important, as there was intense pressure to accept patients whom the unions believed to be dangerous or suicidal and so wished their swift transfer from their workhouses; this was especially so with the London Unions. The committee established the rules and regulations (subject to approval by the Commissioners in Lunacy) for asylum patients and staff, and was also responsible for any maintenance and repairs. They also set the rate charged for the parish paupers, which was agreed at 12 shillings in 1867, which compared favourably with other asylums, such as Norfolk and Cornwall, who charged 14 shillings.[89]

The Committee of Visitors' sixteen members included justices, local dignitaries and several Members of Parliament, as well as the Duke of Northumberland.[90] Some of these doubled up as members of the House Committee (which met on the first and third Fridays of every month) who dealt with the more practical aspects of patient management, for example, the comfort of the new arrivals, patient complaints, as well as ensuring the smooth day-to-day running of the asylum.

Early nineteenth-century concerns regarding wrongful confinement had led to reforming legislation that ensured that private (or paying) patients were certified by independent doctors with no institutional affiliation. Laws regarding the confinement of the insane ensured that there was 'an unfolding system of legal checks and balances', which included a second admission document and a reception order.[91] For pauper patients, the reception order provided a statement of the patient's mental state that was signed by a justice of the peace or a local parish clergyman and authorized by the parish or Poor Law union clerk. For private patients, certification required details of the patient's medical details signed by the petitioner, accompanied by two detailed medical statements that demonstrated the person was of unsound mind, or was an idiot. The documentation provided particulars of the individual's background, status and medical history.

Technically, a pauper was a person whose maintenance was paid for by his or her union or local parish. However, as Bartlett has pointed out, there was contemporary debate as to the actual definition of the pauper within the context of asylum care, as the families of some inmates reimbursed the authorities for the costs of their care.[92] The high numbers of transfers from workhouses to Brookwood suggest many patients would have been on the rolls of the Poor Law prior to admission.[93] Many, whilst not officially labelled as paupers, had relatives who were clearly unable, or unwilling, to pay for their family member's care.

When Brookwood opened, Brushfield reported to the Committee of Visitors that the asylum 'was in a state of forwardness', ready to accept patients as soon as possible 'so as to assist in relieving the urgent requirements of the county'.[94] The transferal of pauper patients from other asylums was a priority; the first admissions on 17 June 1867 were twenty-four patients from the Chertsey and Dorking Unions who had been held in Springfield Asylum, Wandsworth. '[F]rom this date to the end of the year, patients were received as rapidly as was consistent with the proper organisation of a new and large establishment.'[95] Brookwood's patients came from both urban and rural areas of the county although the majority hailed from London during the first twenty-two years. Thereafter, local government reorganization meant more were from rural Surrey. In 1889 the London County Council was formed; this constituted the City of London and twenty-eight metropolitan boroughs, which took in some areas from Middlesex, Surrey and Kent.[96] The largest generators of workhouse patients, parishes such as St Olave's and St Saviour's, for example, were absorbed into these new metropolitan boroughs. This resulted in a substantial shift in the origins and character of the patient profile at Brookwood. Whilst it is not the intention to examine patient data in detail at this point, some statistics are relevant in illustrating Brookwood's general function and location within the provision of lunacy care in nineteenth-century Surrey.

Figure 1.1 shows the total numbers of patients admitted to Brookwood, 1867–97, as well as the numbers of male and female patients admitted each year. Although distribution by sex is discussed later in more detail, it is indicated that the variance in male and female patients was not substantial. In general terms, from 1870 to 1874 all patient admissions were comparatively low, less than two hundred per year, because the asylum was at capacity and the new wings had not yet been completed.[97] The peaks, such as in 1876 (when 451 patients were admitted), and in 1884 (when 585 patients passed through the asylum doors) and again in 1890 is explained by the availability of new accommodation built to meet the relentless demand for places.

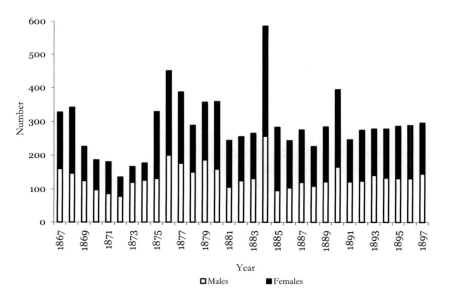

Figure 1.1: Brookwood Asylum, general patient admissions by sex, 1867–97. Source: Patient Admissions Registers, Surrey History Centre.

As highlighted, many patients were transferred from workhouses, the majority of whom were younger, single men, aged sixteen to thirty-five; in some years they accounted for as much as three-quarters of all male admissions. In this age group, a third of these originated from the workhouse, and some from Houses of Correction, compared with only 6 per cent of married men from these institutions. When originally certified, if they were described as dangerous and/or suicidal, they were unable to stay in the workhouse for longer than two weeks, suggesting that these transfers potentially reflected the ability of a particular workhouse to control them.[98] Discipline was always a workhouse priority, and some larger unions, such as Lambeth, built special wards to cater for potentially disruptive young men and women. These were sparsely furnished, with barred windows and doors that could be locked as required. It is probable that overcrowding, and the severity of particular cases, led to a managerial – rather than medical – decision to apply for the transfer of certain pauper lunatics to the asylums.

Historians have shown that workhouses and asylums, in Leicester and in Devon, for example, often co-operated in providing care.[99] But at Brookwood, Brushfield cited the metropolitan unions as being particularly negligent in sending some cases to the asylum, alleging that they were detained for unreasonable periods of time, ostensibly while awaiting the documentation. In their defence, the unions stated that it was the lack of asylum beds that forced them to retain some lunatics; Brushfield was unconvinced, and pointed out that such practices continued even when there was plenty of asylum accommodation available.[100] However, workhouses were keen to transfer their more refractory lunatics, as shown. The workhouses' propensity for delay may have been based upon their desire to retain more biddable patients, being mindful of economy, as opposed to medical considerations, and so they arguably ignored the potential for the individual patient's recovery.

The asylum's records noted many instances of physically ill, dirty and neglected patients arriving from the workhouses. Some bore sores as well as other unexplained marks; some were beyond help. For example, in early 1867, one woman from Bermondsey Workhouse died within seven days of her arrival at Brookwood. Fourteen-year-old Emma M., admitted on 1 September 1871 from St Olave's Workhouse, 'was brought in a decidedly dirty state – her head roaming with vermin. It is evident that during her short residence in the workhouse very little attention was paid to her.'[101] The Brookwood Committee of Visitors recorded and expressed their grave concern at such cases, not all of whom had previously been in workhouse custody. Catherine T., a 32-year-old patient suffering from melancholia, was described as 'very suicidally disposed and maniacal'. She was transferred from Wandsworth to Brookwood completely naked underneath a thick, rough garment resembling a full-length straitjacket complete with locks, straps and gloves, which caused her great distress and obvious physical discomfort. These items were immediately removed when she arrived at Brookwood on 14 July 1871 and were not used again during her stay.[102] The condition of one man removed from his home in 1868 moved Brushfield to report to the Committee:

> One patient, when received, was ascertained to have a severe fracture of the arm, apparently owing to the efforts of the persons who accompanied him (one of them being his own father), to restrain his maniacal excitement during the period of his removal. At the time of his admission his ankles were tied together by a rope, his hands were fastened behind him, and he wore a straightjacket.[103]

These occurrences, which were not unique, suggest that although principles of non-restraint had been generally absorbed into the treatment and handling of the insane within the asylum, the reality for new patients could have been quite different. It was a difficult issue, many patients were distressed and fearful of being moved to new surroundings and resistance could prompt collusion or containment to facilitate their removal.

Admissions to Holloway

The sanatorium was managed by a board of twenty-six trustees, chaired by George Martin Holloway. An annually elected General Committee of between eight and twenty-six members was established, with ex-officio members that included the Trustees, the Lord Lieutenant of Surrey, the Lord Bishop of Winchester, the Lord Mayor of London, the Chairman of the Surrey Quarter Sessions and all the Surrey Justices of the Peace who served as House Committee members of one of the Surrey Asylums. Surrey dignitaries helped the sanatorium become an integral part of the local community, lent gravitas and facilitated charitable donations. Meetings were held twice yearly, although 'Special Meetings' could be instigated at any time if deemed appropriate by the chairman. This committee appointed senior staff members, maintained and audited accounts, and implemented the sanatorium's rules and regulations in accordance with lunacy legislation.

The daily maintenance and housekeeping of the asylum was the responsibility of the House Committee, which met monthly and managed the admissions, regulation of ordinary expenditure, tenders and contracts, as well as overseeing the sanatorium's general and medical administration, and addressing any staff issues. They conducted fortnightly inspections, paying particular attention to the condition and treatment of patients and hearing any complaints. New admissions were subjected to additional scrutiny to ensure correct classification and that appropriate measures for their care and comfort were undertaken. In common with other institutions, including Brookwood, the resident medical superintendent assumed responsibility for the patients' medical treatment and had the 'entire direction of the Institution, subject only to the control of the General and the House Committee'.[104] Supported by two assistant medical officers, the superintendent was responsible for the initial appointment, engagement, regulation and dismissal of all other asylum employees, from the head attendants to the lowest servant.

Holloway patients were intended to be those of the 'middling-sort', and while many suffered from diminished financial circumstances, there is no record of any being directly transferred from workhouses. They were generally in a better physical condition than their Brookwood counterparts, but there were exceptions and some were admitted showing obvious signs of neglect or mistreatment. While charitable assistance was granted to a sizeable number of Holloway's patients, occasionally non-payment of fees necessitated their removal to nearby Brookwood, sometimes with or without the agreement of defaulting relatives.[105]

From the 1880s many advertisements for private nursing homes, sanatoria, inebriate asylums and hydropathic establishments were found in the *Medical Directory*. Aware of middle-class sensitivities to psychiatric illness, Holloway's advertising and brochures advised prospective patients and their families that all correspondence was to be addressed to 'Dr Rees Philipps, Virginia Water, Chertsey', thereby avoiding the term sanatorium.[106] In the same spirit, other institutions altered their name: the licensed house, West Malling Place, previously William Perfect's madhouse, metamorphosed into the Kent Sanatorium.[107] The basic principles that formed the bedrock of the treatment of tuberculosis in nineteenth-century sanatoria, such as fresh air, good diet and controlled exercise, were also much in evidence in the treatment of psychiatric patients. 'Holloway Sanatorium' may thus have helped to preserve middle-class propriety: 'A father will feel terrible repugnance at committing his son to a mad-house, whereas the notion of sending him for a time to a Sanatorium seems far less dreadful'.[108]

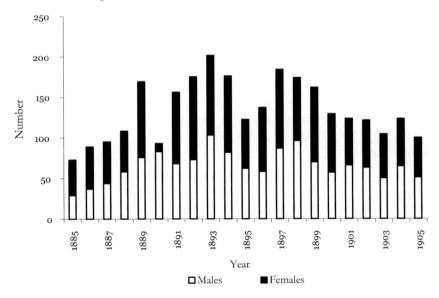

Figure 1.2: Holloway Sanatorium, general patient admissions by sex, 1885–1905, certified patients only. Source: Holloway Admission Registers and Annual Reports, Surrey History Centre.

Similar to Brookwood, the total number of certified patients admitted to the sanatorium between 1885 and 1905 does not reveal any huge disparity between the numbers of male and female admissions. Despite the limitations of the data sample, it can be seen that there were higher numbers admitted in 1893 and 1897 when new patient accommodation was made available to meet the demand for places. Conversely, it can also be seen that in 1890, female admissions in particular were very low due to lack of available beds on the women's side.

Holloway Sanatorium was intended to house 200 patients. It was immediately popular, and within six months there were seventy patients, including eight voluntary boarders. During the course of the following year (1886), eighty-nine certified patients were admitted, plus seventeen boarders. By late 1886, 110 patients and 9 boarders remained. During the first twenty years (1885–1905) a total of 2,815 certified patients and 1,258 voluntary boarders were treated. Overall, women accounted for just over 51 per cent of total admissions during this period, although this was subject to fluctuations and, during the first eighteen months, accounted for as much as 60 per cent (see Figure 1.2).[109] Most female admissions were single women who remained at the sanatorium longer than their male counterparts.[110] This depressed their admission rates, as occasionally the sanatorium simply had no available accommodation for new women patients.

In his first annual report, Dr Philipps remarked that 'several hundreds of applications were received, the greater number expecting to be admitted gratuitously or at a low rate of board'.[111] The management opined that such admissions had to be restricted. Despite sufficient patient income, in 1886 the General Committee was reluctant to admit too many highly subsidized cases, as they were detrimental to the hospital's financial well-being. In addition, subsidies encouraged the admission of an unhealthy number of incurable cases. In spite of their caution, the House Committee endeavoured to acknowledge the sanatorium's original philanthropic intentions, and admitted sixty-eight patients at reduced rates.

> The benevolent object with which the Institution was founded has not been lost sight of. Several patients, including one kept gratuitously, have been maintained at low weekly rates ... Indirect aid has also been given to certain patients in the shape of clothing and other extras.[112]

Applications for assisted rates were usually made by patients' relatives and friends, but occasionally by the patients themselves, especially the voluntary boarders. These applications were then considered at General Committee meetings, where personal recommendations from committee members more favourably considered, as were applications from former members of the armed forces, diplomatic services, the medical profession and clergy. The patient's familial, social and occupational status was evaluated to ensure that the applicants were 'of the middling sort'.

How the committee arrived at their decisions to support these applications is unclear from the records, and there is no evidence of a consistent criterion being applied.[113] The Hospital Rules for the Admission and Visiting of Patients and Boarders in 1889 stated that fees varied from £2.2s. to £3.3s. per week and that reductions for special cases were entirely at the discretion of the committee.[114] Patients and their representatives were allowed to make personal, as opposed to written, appeals to the committee. As Wright has also demonstrated for the county asylum in Buckinghamshire, the confinement process was frequently a collaboration between patients' families and the hospital management, with the superintendent playing a contributory, as opposed to a pivotal, role in the admissions process.[115]

Class definitions within asylums more generally are fraught with ambiguities. Lorraine Walsh's work on the Dundee Royal Lunatic Asylum (with its separate private patient facility), showed that respectability and social propriety were important determinants in patient selection for admission.[116] Respectability in Victorian Britain was defined as a way of living that embodied morals, morality and financial prudence that was usually accompanied by independence. Life could be hard, but those who were brought low through no fault of their own, and who still retained their self-respect, were worthy of admiration, and ultimately, assistance.[117] At Holloway, only those patients meeting the board's 'criteria' were considered worthy of charitable assistance. Just as some of Brookwood's patients were not paupers, so, too, some patients at Holloway were of 'scanty means'. As the century drew to a close, more upper-class admissions were allowed to subsidize them. The ambiguities of class and social tensions of position have been examined by Joseph Melling in relation to governess patients, who were admitted to both private and public asylums.[118] It was patients such as these who applied for reduced fees upon admission to Holloway, some with a degree of success.[119]

Prior to opening, the intention was that patients would be allowed to stay at the sanatorium for a maximum of one year, so that the institution would be seen as a temporary refuge for afflicted members of the impoverished middle classes. An anonymous article in the *Builder* in 1882 (probably written by Godwin), noted the 'novel' conditions and rules that Thomas Holloway set for his sanatorium, which '[is] not intended to be devoted to the uses of an ordinary asylum for the insane'.[120] All patients were to be middle class. In addition:

> no patient will be allowed to remain an inmate of the institution for a longer period than twelve months; no patient will be received whose case is considered hopeless; no patient will be allowed to enter the Sanatorium after having been once discharged.[121]

These rules were similar to those initially issued by other institutions, such as Bethlem and St Luke's, but all were obliged to relax their restrictions over time.[122]

Many patients were readmitted to Holloway, and cases such as that of Eva A. were not unique. Religious and identity delusions beset this 21-year-old Hampstead woman and, in 1898, following a brief stay at a private licensed house in Hendon, she was admitted to Holloway as a voluntary boarder. She remained as such for six months, before being discharged in July 1899. Over the next five years, she was admitted to Holloway on five separate occasions, initially as a voluntary boarder in most cases, but was always subsequently certified within days. She was finally discharged as recovered in October 1905, and at no point in her records were there any apparent difficulties regarding her many readmissions.[123]

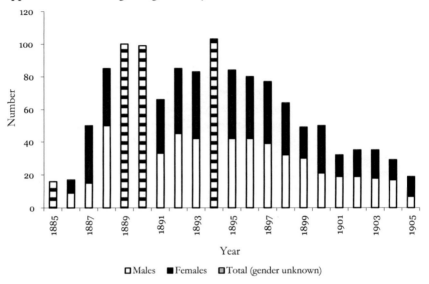

Figure 1.3: Holloway Sanatorium, general patient admissions by sex, 1885–1905, voluntary boarders only. Source: Holloway Admissions Registers and Annual Reports, Surrey History Centre.

The data in Figure 1.3 shows the admissions to Holloway Sanatorium over the 21-year period from 1885 to 1905 for one specific class of patient only – the voluntary boarders. This arguably less formalized approach to entering the sanatorium did not require certification for patients to utilize the facilities and to be medically treated. The record-keeping for these patients was less thorough, which may have contributed to the fact that there is missing admissions data for some years, as seen in Figure 1.3 for the years 1889–90 and 1894.

Little attention has been paid by historians to the voluntary system.[124] Voluntary admissions to Holloway accounted for 31 per cent of all admissions during the period from 1885 to 1905, but declined as a percentage of total admissions after 1898. Annual reports frequently testified to the medical staff's belief that the voluntary boarder system assisted both patient well-being and the efficacy of treatment. Non-certification minimized stigma and, as such, removed a perceived hindrance to the recovery process. Many of these patients were subsequently certified, but this was by no means always the case. Readmissions and prolonged periods of residence were marked amongst the voluntary boarders. Information has been particularly difficult to extrapolate, due to the limited extant records. What has survived is often inconsistent and patchy for the voluntary patients.

The voluntary system allowed patients with less serious conditions to be admitted for respite care. Helen W. was first admitted in August 1891 at the request of her mother. A young, single, epileptic woman, she was described as being 'weak-minded', however, 'she answers questions rationally, recognises money value, understands the chief political events of the day, and appears to have a good memory. Though unable to earn her living does not appear a suitable subject for certification.'[125] During the following fourteen months, she was admitted under voluntary status on five occasions, notably when suffering many fits on a daily basis which her family were unable to cope with. This admission pattern was repeated several times during the following eight years.

The 1886 regulations described three categories of patients admissible to the Holloway Sanatorium, whether or not they were certified or boarders. These were: curable patients who were unable to pay at all; patients either curable or incurable who could not afford full payment; and patients, whether curable or incurable, whose circumstances did allow for full payment.[126] First class rates were set at £2.2s. and upward, and second class at between £1.5s. and £2.2s. Rates of payment for both the third class and urgent second class cases were determined by the medical superintendent and then submitted for approval by the House Committee. Gratuitous admissions and maintenance cases, whether boarder or patient, had to be approved by the House Committee in the first instance, and were intended only for those patients deemed to have a high probability of being cured.[127]

In 1889 the hospital was registered as a charity. Thereafter, a minimum of 50 per cent of admissions had to be accommodated at a weekly inclusive rate not exceeding two guineas, and a quarter of all admissions for 25 shillings or less.[128] This was supplemented by other patients, so that by 1891, 28 per cent of patients occupied the more substantial first-class accommodation at the front of the institution, paying over 42 shillings per week. Here they enjoyed private rooms, often with special attendants, or, if their relatives preferred, they could be accommodated in a private cottage in the grounds. Most patients, 45 per cent, were 'second class', paying between 42 and 25 shillings per week, with the remaining 27 per cent of third-class patients on rates of 25 shillings or less.[129] By 1891 the hospital's charitable aid was over £4,000 and was 'mainly bestowed on patients of good social position but scanty means, who could not obtain equal comforts in private asylums, except at greatly increased cost'.[130] At the request of the hospital's management, charitable assistance was extended to include the much-favoured voluntary boarders.

Ensuring that patients met the criteria of 'middle class' was problematic for the asylum's management and, realistically, the term must have retained some variability. It is clear that the middling sort formed the core of the patients, but it was financially expedient, for example, that high ranking and, therefore usually higher fee-paying patients were also admitted, either as volunteers or under certification. Some Chancery lunatics were resident and, with a guaranteed income from the trustees of their estates, helped balance the asylum's books.[131] In addition, a very small number of criminal lunatics were admitted, usually those who had been incarcerated for relatively petty offences and had served their time.

The Daily Routine

The asylum's medical regime was established by the medical superintendent with the assistance of his chief medical officers, but within a standard format that strove to instil order and security for the benefit of patients and staff alike.[132] The quality of life for all was affected by rapid growth in numbers, the attendant building work at both asylums, and shifts in medical priorities. Although increased numbers of inmates influenced this shift, it also reflected developments in both medical perceptions and advancements. As a pauper asylum, Brookwood had to provide a secure and therapeutic environment for a large number of patients in a cost-effective way. The days were long: the asylum day began at 6 am and during waking hours, day in, and day out, patients had to be kept meaningfully employed to ensure their manageability. They suffered from a range of mental and physical disabilities of varying degrees of acuteness or chronicity. Where appropriate, suitable patients were put to work, and the various activities and entertainments that were incorporated into the asylum's calendar were made available to all but the most infirm or ungovernable.

Brookwood patients thus had a varied programme of entertainment and activities. Private asylums, for example Ticehurst or charitable institutions such as St Luke's, frequently organized excursions, balls and dances, as their better class of inmate was perceived to require some form of physical exertion and occupation that did not centre on manual labour. To a lesser extent, public asylums, such as the one at Denbigh, also provided amusements, especially during the summer months, when the annual ball was the highlight of the social calendar.[133] Initially, such asylum activities aroused public curiosity in general society, but they were soon generally accepted.[134] In 1875, the *Surrey Advertiser* commented that Dr Brushfield had for many years endeavoured to familiarize observers with the notion of 'intellectual entertainments', such as those which he had organized previously during his time as superintendent at Chester Asylum. These entertainments, including theatricals, formed a core component in his treatment of the patients, and he believed they assisted their recovery process and the return to normal life. Through participation and observation of such social occasions, patients were offered the opportunity to exhibit rationality and social competence, which in turn could lead them to rehabilitation in society. As such, the entertainments were a component of moral treatment and thus a humane reintroduction into the many aspects of everyday life. Such interactions in social activities within the local community also suggest that some institutions were not as isolated as may have been originally intended as therapeutic perspectives altered.

To relieve the monotony of asylum life, a weekly entertainment of readings, concerts, conjuring shows, marionettes or pantomimes was enacted. On alternate weeks, a ball allowed male and female patients the opportunity to associate and participate in the dancing; the first was held on 19 September 1867 and was attended by over three-quarters of the patients.[135] Over the years, as the numbers of inmates grew, entertainments were restricted, but walks for the patients became a regular feature, as they were free and required close supervision for a relatively short period of time. Occasionally these took place beyond the grounds for some well-behaved patients, but the Commissioners in Lunacy were disappointed to note that up to a quarter of the male patients exercised only within the airing courts.[136]

Cards and games such as draughts and dominoes were supplied to all wards. The Committee of Visitors approved of efforts made to enliven the environment, including suitable reading material, and that 'objects of interests such as framed pictures, birds, etc. are gradually being added. The cheaper forms of illustrated periodicals are regularly circulated, and a library is being instituted. A brass band is also being formed.'[137] The frequent replenishment of these prompted the Committee of Visitors to seek donations of cards, books, games and pictures and other items; for example, in 1867 they appealed to their members for a piano for the entertainment of female patients.[138]

The *Surrey Advertiser* observed that, whilst asylum entertainments were no longer novel, they were always 'interesting', not least because it was possible to observe a 'lunatic audience conducting itself well' and also to perceive the level of artistic skills revealed by such performances.[139] The balls appeared to have offered the greatest entertainment of all. 'Besides, it is cheering to the onlookers to witness the vivacious movements contrasting with uncouth and well intentioned antics meant for dancing, by a few who would do better if they could.'[140] These occasions suggest that Brookwood Asylum became part of the local community; the audiences at the theatricals, for example, 'contained a large number of ladies and gentlemen from the surrounding county', in particular doctors, ministers of the cloth 'and the County Surveyor'.[141]

Amusements existed for the relief of the employees, too. Caring for the insane was perceived as a demanding and often unpleasant job, so that finding and retaining good attendants was difficult for asylum superintendents. Often attendants were young and single and lived on the premises. They had limited free time and were somewhat isolated. At Brookwood, members of staff at all levels were not merely organizers, but frequently were active participants in the asylum's dances and sporting events. Skills in both music and sports were seen as vital constituents of the potential attendant's personal attributes. The asylum's brass band played at local fêtes and events, and there were regular cricket and football fixtures where inmates competed against other custodial institutions, and where the staff frequently participated. Such events went some way to alleviating the tedium of life for attendants, who lived for much of their time isolated in the asylum, and were liable to become almost as institutionalized as the patients.

Unlike the nearby Holloway Sanatorium whose largely middle-class clientele were unused to manual labour and where appropriate behaviour and manners were emphasized, Brookwood's daily regime incorporated a rigorous work schedule. This ensured both therapy and occupation for the patients whilst also helping the asylum to maintain some self-sufficiency. In turn, it provided a degree of normalization, in that the strategy had the potential for retraining patients and building a work ethic that would, it was hoped, reduce or even remove their reliance on poor relief once they were discharged.[142] Brookwood's location had been partially chosen as the size of the land enabled patients to work on an asylum farm. As at other asylums, the gains were perceived to be in moral treatment, in institutional self-sufficiency and in helping financial viability. The Commissioners in Lunacy, reporting on their visit to Brookwood in November 1868, observed with satisfaction that 133 male and 180 female patients were being 'usefully employed'. Gender divisions were evident in employment. Of the men, seventy worked on the land, whilst twenty were employed as tailors, shoemakers, painters and bricklayers. The remainder helped in the wards, or as coal carriers. Of the women, twenty-seven toiled in the ever-busy laundry, eight in the kitchen, some forty to fifty were cleaners, and others were employed in sewing, knitting, netting or bookbinding.[143] Whilst all the patient work contributed to the asylum's drive for self-sufficiency, the men's labour in food provision was seen as of particular value.

The superintendent reported in 1869 that an average of two-thirds of the patients were employed and, although a few men were occupied in the artisan's workshops, most worked outdoors. Importantly, this allowed for the gradual cultivation of many acres of previously barren and sandy heath, so that it became possible to grow oats, rye, barley, potatoes and turnips. Brushfield reported that the kitchen garden yielded ample green vegetables for the consumption of the asylum population, and further, that within two years of opening, livestock provided the kitchen with 3,215 gallons of milk and 1,114 stones of pork.[144]

From a therapeutic perspective, the comfort and elegance available to Holloway patients was designed to ease their adjustment to their changed circumstances, whilst the 'normality' of a homely but luxurious environment was believed to be beneficial to recovery. This concern to preserve 'normality' was an ongoing consideration for the medical superintendent and governors. With the spread of the railway network, seaside trips were popular and had become part of many Victorian families' itineraries.[145] In addition, the management believed in the therapeutic value of fresh air and so rented coastal properties for the use of their patients during the summer months. Eventually, they purchased their own property at Hove and later, a larger property at Canford Cliffs, Dorset.[146] Similarly, St Luke's Hospital acquired a second property in 1898 at St Lawrence-on-Sea, near Ramsgate, which was used for a small number of female convalescents. Brookwood did not have the advantage of a seaside residence, nor of temporarily moving groups of patients to another therapeutic environment. Cost was, of course, a consideration, and although seemingly rare, other public asylums, such as Devon, sought this type of short-term arrangement.[147]

'Of the greatest use in promoting occupation and amusement' were the companions employed at Holloway to live amongst the patients and encourage normal behaviour and conversation.[148] These middle-class employees were generally not required to perform nursing duties. Initially, there were two males and two females, although between six and nine companions were engaged on each side of the house most years. Their daily duties included eating with the patients, ensuring they were appropriately dressed, accompanying them on walks and participating in various recreational amusements such as embroidery, bagatelle or cards. They also helped the superintendent and assistant medical officers to plan and execute the entertainment schedule. Overall, the companions were seen as a valuable asset to the resocialization and training of the Holloway patients. However, things did not always run smoothly and, just like asylum attendants, they did break the rules, as in the case of Mr Mayne, one of the male companions, who was removed from his post following a bout of intemperance.[149]

Entertainment was an important component of Holloway's therapeutic regime, and the patients were able to participate in a full and varied programme of activities and social events. This is partly attributable to the fact that the alternative of physical labour was not appropriate for the majority of patients. This contrasted with Brookwood, where all patients were expected to be usefully employed, unless sickness or age prevented them.[150] The programme of amusements would also have encouraged bourgeois patients to come to the sanatorium, since Holloway's varied recreation rivalled that of Ticehurst Asylum in its scope, although admittedly the Sussex institution offered additional facilities such as 'hunting with harriers' which was seen as a suitable occupation for its upper-class patients.[151] George Martin Holloway, writing a draft biography of his brother-in-law's life, stated that the intention was to provide 'all the elegancies of a refined House'.[152] Tennis courts (flooded in the winter for skating), billiards rooms, a cricket and football pitch, and a swimming pool in the summer months, were all available for the patient's use. Archery, golf and croquet were regularly played, and by 1894 a gym was available for male patients who were trained in Swedish drill.[153]

There was an extensive range of recreational facilities. There were classes in oils, watercolours, drawing, photography and needlework, with the results proudly displayed in exhibitions. There was a well-stocked library, as well as visits from brass bands, choirs and theatrical groups. Other activities recorded in the superintendent's annual reports included picnics, cricket matches, garden parties, outdoor fêtes, dances, music and dinner parties, excursions to the seaside or to London, as well as shopping trips. Some wealthier patients attended local social events and ventured out on river excursions. Whilst Rees Philipps bemoaned the lack of a London property for patients to stay and avail themselves of the capital's varied amusements, this was never a serious consideration for the General Committee and it did not seem to have had an adverse effect on the patients or on the sanatorium's reputation. Some of the more affluent and able patients were entrusted to organize their own independent social life, assisted by their private servants; so many maintained their own carriage and pair at the sanatorium that additional stabling had to be built.[154] For lower middle-class patients, it may be supposed that they experienced a better lifestyle than they had known prior to admission; this possibly contributed to the decision of many medically discharged patients to stay on at Holloway on a voluntary basis.

It is perhaps surprising that many patients were entrusted with a substantial amount of freedom, partially due to the superintendent's deference to their social class and also as there was always a high proportion of voluntary patients. The superintendent steadfastly maintained this policy, despite occasional abuses of trust and some evidence that this liberty enabled patients to continue with their destructive habits. Some would visit nearby shops to make prohibited purchases, and a few ventured into local public houses where they became such a nuisance that they had to be removed forcibly by attendants. Occasionally, the pre-agreed excursions lasted considerably longer than had been decided and there were several occurrences of patients venturing beyond the restricted three-mile radius of the hospital, often disappearing for days. One such case was a gentleman boarder who was eventually traced and found wandering on Derby racecourse, an incident that incurred the condemnation of the Commissioners in Lunacy regarding the care and control of the sanatorium's voluntary patients.

Conclusion

Unlike the glorious, but initially impractical, buildings of Holloway Sanatorium, Brookwood Asylum was a comparatively plain, functional institution that reflected the need to spend ratepayers' money frugally. The sanatorium's modern facilities enabled relatively small numbers of largely middle-class patients to benefit from a therapeutic environment that offered a vast array of activities and entertainment. In contrast, Brookwood, as a much larger county asylum, battled with ever-increasing demands for admission, which in turn generated tensions between 'care and custody'. In common with other county pauper asylums at the time, the management of the county's lunatics was influenced by the policies of local Poor Law officials, although Brookwood opposed pressure for increased admissions and highlighted the condition of patients transferred from workhouses. But, unlike some other pauper asylums, where bureaucratic and financial constraints meant that therapies (moral, chemical and physical) decreased, the Brookwood management did successfully strive to elevate the asylum's status beyond that of a merely custodial institution, and to expand the range of patients' occupation and exercise.[155]

In describing the late nineteenth-century world of the middle-class and/or deserving recipient of charitable mental health care within an environment specifically created for them at Holloway, this chapter has shown how this world differed from that of the pauper inmate at Brookwood. This was despite the fact that the middle-class and the pauper insane suffered from the same illnesses which ultimately required some form of long-term care and therapeutics. Where indicated, the causes of the illness were more likely to vary and were reflective of many contemporary class-based contexts and concerns. This chapter has thus begun to explore the differentiated class-based patient experience of the asylum which will be analysed further throughout the book.

2 THERAPEUTIC AGENTS: DOCTORS AND ATTENDANTS

Introduction

The successful functioning of any private or public nineteenth-century asylum largely depended on reliable, caring staff at all levels, and this chapter will explore how Brookwood Asylum and Holloway Sanatorium utilized their attendants and other employees to their best advantage. From the superintendent, his medical officers, attendants, nurses and the chaplain, to the maids and the cook, the gardeners and the lowliest servants, all contributed to the efficient daily running of institutions that required strict routine and continuity of service. At both asylums, the first medical superintendents and their supporting officers held their posts for relatively long periods of time which provided stability; arguably, they also imposed their beliefs and personal styles upon the daily routines and the implementation of any therapeutic regime. Asylums experienced difficulties in recruiting and retaining good attendants; once employed, the management's strategy of monitoring and regulating their staff in order to maintain standards will be discussed and measured. The middle-class patients at Holloway meant that at this sanatorium some specific staffing strategies were employed in order to satisfy the expectations of the inmates and their families. It also becomes apparent that despite the many rigours of institutional life, asylum nursing did offer security of employment for many, and career opportunities for some.

By the mid-nineteenth century, the descriptive term 'mad-doctor' had all but disappeared from common parlance. From the 1860s, the term 'alienist' was more commonly applied to the medical superintendent or resident medical officer, but it also referred to any medical professional who specialized in the treatment of the mentally unsound.[1] The term 'psychiatry' appeared in Europe and by 1910 this term and associated ones (psychiatric, psychiatrist) were widely used and associated with the professional care of insanity and lesser mental disorders.[2] The middle and upper classes increasingly sought help for their mentally distressed relatives, and these clients arguably raised the social and medical status of some practitioners; nevertheless, asylum-based medicine remained firmly stigmatized. Caring for the insane was not considered a good career choice, as there was a perceived lack of professionalism, endorsed by the lack of available formalized training. Marginalized by the mainstream medical profession, the superintendent of a sprawling county institution was unlikely to be considered on a par with a colleague at a teaching hospital or a prestigious university.

Legislative changes expanded the county asylum network, and caring for the mad became increasingly regulated as general recognition grew of the need for professionalization in this field. The Association of Medical Officers of Hospitals for the Insane was formed in 1841 in order to raise the professional status, and thus obtain medical and general acceptability. In 1853 the organization was renamed the Association of Medical Officers of Asylums and Hospitals for the Insane, which was felt to be more reflective of their members' origin, before it was changed again in 1865 to become the Medico-Psychological Association.[3] As Oppenheim has pointed out, these titular alterations (also reflected in the publication of their journal) clearly were designed to raise awareness that mental disorders were not merely confined to asylums and lunatics, but that they belonged to the wider catalogue of medical diseases, and so were accessible by scientific inquiry in the same way.[4]

The Medico-Psychological Association sought to alter popular (and largely unfavourable) perceptions of asylum workers by providing educational initiatives for all levels of staff to enhance their professional image. Early efforts were limited to a few medical schools that offered restricted clinical instruction on a voluntary basis. However, during the 1860s and 1870s, there were increased calls for the compulsory inclusion of lectures on mental diseases within the medical undergraduate curriculum. From 1885, the Association began to encourage asylum doctors to sit for its own newly established Certificate of Efficiency in Psychological Medicine.[5] By 1890 the General Medical Council ensured that psychological medicine was included for both study and examination. Despite the inclusion of mental diseases and their treatment in medical training, it remained a comparatively small component until the First World War, and asylum doctors continued to be somewhat marginalized by the rest of their profession.[6]

Asylum Doctors

The 1845 Asylum Act led to an increase in the provision of county and borough asylums that were to be regularly inspected by the Commissioners in Lunacy, who were empowered to visit any institution that accommodated lunatics. Amongst the many new practices that asylums were obliged to adopt, was the regular maintenance of detailed records and medical case books that clearly recorded the details of each patient's illness and their subsequent treatment. This practice emphasized the importance of medical care and specialization within the context of the asylum, which paved the way for new medical positions for qualified medical practitioners at these institutions.

The most important member of the asylum staff was the medical superintendent, whose personal and professional style characterized the institution, albeit within the constraints of ever-increasing bureaucratic accountability and medical specialization. It has been suggested that medical superintendents tended to run the asylums in a patriarchal manner, although their control was delegated through assistant doctors (or medical officers), who assumed the day-to-day responsibility for the patients' medical care.[7] The large number of Brookwood's inmates certainly necessitated such delegation, although the unexpectedly high volume of admissions at both asylums meant that it was necessary to recruit more staff almost immediately after opening. In addition to assistant medical officers, the superintendent hired male and female attendants, as well as a chaplain, domestic and ancillary staff and, in the case of Holloway, male and female companions. Once employed, the staff became isolated in predominantly rural environments, with few opportunities for offsite recreational diversion.

Both institutions benefited from the long service of their first medical superintendents, which provided consistency and stability. Whilst details of their daily routines are largely unknown, the superintendents' contributions to annual reports and specialist journals, in addition to colleagues' testimonials, provide some evidence of how each asylum bore the stamp of their respective managers.[8] The superintendent's role encompassed both medical and administrative tasks, with the latter becoming increasingly demanding as legislative changes occurred which were accompanied by increased official scrutiny. Brookwood was more bureaucratic, being answerable to the Commissioners in Lunacy, Poor Law officials, local government and ratepayers.[9] Aside from supervising patients and managing staff, the superintendent routinely reported to the House Committee and the Committee of Visitors.

As a result of its charitable status acquired in 1889, Holloway's superintendent was not only accountable to the Commissioners in Lunacy but also to the Charities Commission. Since the hospital was independent, with a high number of fee-paying patients, there was the additional responsibility of satisfying patients' families and relatives, whose social status made them both articulate and demanding. Additional administrative work arose from the many applications received for subsidized fees as the sanatorium's management strove to maintain its philanthropic ideals. Since a considerable number of patients were granted charitable assistance, more work for the superintendent could result from patients' families' refusal (or inability) to pay the residual fees, necessitating additional engagement with the Poor Law authorities.

Brookwood was obliged to expand rapidly; by 1900 there were 1,050 inmates, swelling to 1,750 by 1938. Such growth was not uncommon.[10] Brookwood's first superintendent, Dr Brushfield, prioritized the safe and efficient organization of all classes of patients, whilst attempting to 'cure' as many as possible. By contrast, Holloway opened with accommodation for 200 patients, although its popularity meant that it, too, grew quickly. By 1894, the number of residents had almost doubled to 394, and remained roughly at this level until 1905.[11] Brookwood's first Medical Superintendent was Thomas Nadauld Brushfield MD (1828–1910). After a period at the London Hospital as Resident House-Surgeon, he gained experience at Bethnal House Asylum before spending fourteen years at Chester County Asylum.[12] He was appointed at Brookwood shortly before opening, primarily in an advisory capacity to ensure all was correct and ready to receive the patients.[13] Poor Law officials hailed this new Surrey asylum as the solution to the problem of the county's increasingly numerous pauper insane, and, as preparations for opening were made, south London parishes exerted great pressure to transfer large numbers of insane inmates from their workhouses. Brushfield responded by imposing restrictions to ensure that the asylum was not overrun with patients who were either in a very poor mental and physical condition, or were incurable, or both. He believed that too many patients of this type inhibited the efficacy of medical treatment for those who were likely to recover. His reports show that this was a continual problem throughout his tenure, but they also demonstrate his firm commitment to the care of both his patients and staff, despite the sheer weight of numbers. Although the treatment regime and system adopted at Brookwood was fairly widely practised in asylums by this time, Brushfield's interpretation of moral therapy was still viewed by contemporaries as innovative.[14] 'He was a first-rate asylum superintendent', said his obituary in the *British Medical Journal*, 'and practically introduced a new era in the treatment of the insane'.[15] Physically attacked by patients on at least two occasions, he ran Brookwood for nearly seventeen years until he was forced to retire following a serious assault by an inmate.[16]

Brushfield emphasized the value of occupation as well as entertainment that often engaged with the local community.[17] Although not a novel approach, moral therapy encompassed a broad range of non-medical treatments which involved the patient in his or her recovery process, so that the patient gained sufficient self-mastery to overcome illness.[18] Strongly associated with the York Retreat, a more humane and collaborative approach was in evidence at institutions such as Conolly's Hanwell Asylum, as well as being practised in Philippe Pinel's Parisian hospitals. To attempt to relieve insanity, the focus was on the psychological or emotional faculties of the patients. The interpretation of moral treatment that evolved in the larger asylums, and its juxtaposition with emergent theories of physical or hereditary causality, mean that it was obliged to adapt and change over time.[19] Praised for his 'intelligent application of practices of non-restraint' and the minimal cases of seclusion, Brushfield was known not to dogmatize, nor did he 'condemn those who differ from him and discredit his system of treatment'.[20] His reports openly highlighted the common difficulties of running a large institution, yet he largely avoided pessimism, and engaged in matters of contemporary debate and interest as described above. Alienists, or asylum doctors, have latterly been accused of seeking professionalization as a component of blatant self-interest (see for example, the work of Andrew Scull).[21] But Brushfield's reputation and his continual efforts to find more effective means of caring for and curing his patients, do not substantiate this view.

Naturally, the administration of the asylum was burdensome. Almost immediately after Brookwood opened, an assistant medical officer was engaged to alleviate the ever-increasing clinical and administrative responsibilities. The first in post, Francis Skae, only stayed nine months and was succeeded by Edward Swain, who left after four years (1874) to become superintendent of Three Counties Asylum, Arlesey. The next officer, James Barton, was promoted in 1882 to become Brookwood's second medical superintendent; he remained in this post for the next twenty-three years.[22] The long careers of asylum superintendents, although beneficial in some respects, arguably could inhibit the professional advancement of capable assistant medical officers, who were poorly enumerated and socially isolated.[23] In this light, Barton's eight-year apprenticeship was a comparatively short one. From 1875, more patient admissions made it necessary to employ a second assistant medical officer, a post briefly occupied initially by William Thomson, who was succeeded a year later by James Moody, formally of St Luke's Hospital. He left Brookwood in 1882 and at the age of twenty-nine became superintendent of the new Cane Hill Asylum, where he remained until his death, thirty-three years later.[24]

Dr Sutherland Rees Philipps (1848–1925) was the first medical superintendent at Holloway Sanatorium, where he remained in service for fifteen years.[25] During his general medical training, he had become increasingly interested in mental illness, and after holding a series of hospital appointments, he joined the Devon County Asylum and then moved to the Three Counties Asylum as senior assistant medical officer. Later he was appointed medical superintendent to the private Wonford House Hospital, Exeter, before coming to Holloway.[26] He too was engaged some time prior to the sanatorium's official opening (from 1884), as there were many legal and structural problems that had prevented it from being licensed, and for which he then assumed responsibility. In the months leading up to the official opening, he personally engaged the architects and builders, and oversaw the works to a satisfactory completion.

Additional administrative pressures came from the hospital's charitable status, and the many applications for reduced patient fees. Similarly, managing the high numbers of the sanatorium's voluntary admissions (uncertified patients) was not straightforward. This practice was frowned upon by the Commissioners in Lunacy, but the superintendent believed that admitting patients under a voluntary banner minimized the associated stigma, and so aided the recovery process.[27] Rees Philipps's role was further complicated by the need to seek a compromise between appropriate treatment and middle-class propriety.[28] Class-based tensions affected certain aspects of the sanatorium's daily management, including the recruitment of appropriate attendants and nurses and the difficulties that could arise from boarders and patients being instructed by their social inferiors. In order to address this tension, Rees Philipps employed lady and gentlemen companions, and he appointed his wife to manage Holloway's seaside branch at Hove (1892–1909) which provided holidays and convalescence for the sanatorium patients. Mrs Philipps was listed in local trade directories as the female superintendent, and she took a particular pride in running this branch, personally supervising its daily routine and choosing to live amongst the patients as opposed to occupying separate quarters.[29]

Both voluntary and certified patients were entitled to apply for charitable assistance and, by 1891, two-thirds of the patients were in receipt of some level of support. The remainder paid full rates for the very best accommodation that the sanatorium could offer, often bringing with them their own servants, horses and coaches for the duration. These wealthier patients were demanding, expecting deference from all around them, but although exacting, they made a vital financial contribution to the sanatorium's finances. Rees Philipps acknowledged their importance, their status and their value. In addition to addressing other social issues, the fit were allowed to attend days out during the Season as a concession and he tried to secure more appropriate social facilities for them (such as a seaside home and a house in central London).

Rees Philipps was helped by his assistant medical officer, Dr Moynan, who joined in August 1885 and remained in post until 1888.[30] That year, the increased patient numbers led to the decision to engage a temporary assistant medical officer for several months before Mr C. H. Dixon was appointed permanently. Rees Philipps was delighted with the new recruit, reporting the 'kindly and sympathetic way in which he cared for the patients under his charge'.[31] Thereafter, the superintendent was assisted by a senior and a junior medical officer on both the male and female sides. The next senior assistant medical officer was Dr A. N. Little, and Dr Charles Caldecott was engaged as junior assistant medical officer (both were appointed in 1889).[32] Given their Poor Law institution background, they may have been anxious to escape the associated stigma, as well as benefiting from a more convivial environment. However, Little eventually found his sanatorium duties too stressful and, after nearly five years' service, he resigned in 1894 'on the ground of being unable longer to contend with the worries and cares of asylum life'.[33] Following the retirement of Rees Philipps, Dr William David Moore was appointed his successor, having successfully deputized at both Virginia Water and the Hove branch during his predecessor's illness.[34]

Until the end of the nineteenth century, asylum doctors were predominantly male; female doctors were not admitted to the Medico-Psychological Association until 1893. Anne Digby has commented that, as medical expertise grew, women were increasingly reduced to a subordinate role, and that 'female authority was not to be revived until women had themselves trained as doctors'.[35] At the York Retreat, Norah Kemp was the first female assistant medical officer, appointed in 1889.[36] Women who worked in asylums generally occupied supportive and lesser positions, such as nurses and domestic servants. The matron was the most senior position amongst the female staff, aside from the superintendent's wife, who may or may not have taken an active role in the daily running of the asylum; whilst little is known about Mrs Brushfield's activities at Brookwood, as shown, Mrs Rees Philipps took an active role. She was not the only doctor's wife employed at Holloway; Mrs Caldecott, who reputedly excelled in sport and music, worked as a charge nurse on the female side until her husband was appointed superintendent at Earlswood Asylum in 1896.[37]

Psychiatry generally had a low status within the medical profession, and so it was one area that was receptive to employing newly qualified women doctors.[38] There were no female doctors at Brookwood in the nineteenth century, but in the 1890s, Dr Rees Philipps employed three women as medical officers at Holloway. His receptiveness to this relatively new trend is perhaps in keeping with his view of the advantages of employing women to care for the insane middle classes. But although their contribution was valued, they were never entirely viewed as equal to their male counterparts. The first female doctor to be employed at Holloway was Jane B. Henderson, junior medical officer, who worked with the female patients from 1 October 1890. She also had a background in obstetrics.[39] The superintendent explained his decision by commenting that 'The addition of a qualified medical woman to the staff has enabled due attention to be paid to a class of diseases which are often neglected in the routine of Asylum work'.[40] These may have been conditions specifically associated with women at that time, such as types of hysteria, or auto-erotic inclinations, which may have caused mutual embarrassment to patients and staff. Henderson was replaced in September 1893 by Emily Louisa Dove, who left in December 1895 to become assistant medical officer at the London County Asylum at Claybury.[41] Rees Philipps reported to the General Committee that 'She has always done her work in a very conscientious and efficient way, and I was very sorry to lose her'. Rosina Clara Despard MB,[42] 'whose distinguished career at London University and evident enthusiasm for work give promise that she will be a valuable officer',[43] was the next female doctor to be employed at Holloway. As junior assistant medical officer from January 1896, on the female side, she fulfilled all of Rees Philipps's expectations, and remained a valued member of staff until 1909. These female doctors consolidated Rees Philipps's statement that the 'experience of female medical officers convinces me that they are valuable auxiliaries and almost indispensable to any asylum'.[44]

In order to secure the smooth running of asylums, firm boundaries between the patients and the medical staff had to be established and respected. The first stage of this process was the patients' acceptance of the medical superintendent's authority, and that of the other doctors and staff. Attendants and nurses were important not only in the medical and practical sense, but also in that their demeanour, behaviour and even their social skills were believed to have a profound influence on their charges. The asylum management demanded high personal and moral standards in its staff and dealt with any transgressions firmly and quickly.

The scope and type of treatments available within each asylum, to some degree, may have varied according to the philosophy of the medical superintendent, although economic factors also influenced the frequency of chemical intervention and the adoption (or not) of new therapies. The annual reports and the patients' case books provide some evidence of the treatment and care.[45] They also give some insight into the ethos that underpinned the therapeutic regimes which were occasionally discussed in more depth by the superintendents, in articles submitted to specialist journals. At Brookwood and Holloway, the first superintendents provided many years of leadership, consistency and stability to their particular regimes. Both medical men would have shared similar concerns, not least the engagement and maintenance of suitable asylum attendants, which were vital for the security and well-being of the patients as well as the asylum's reputation.

Asylum Attendants

Although maintaining custody and security was crucial in the asylum, particularly with the rise of the non-restraint movement and the implementation of moral treatment, attendants were increasingly viewed as therapeutic agents.[46] The attendants implemented the superintendent's directives and all aspects of the therapeutic regime, which was especially important when it came to the care of suicidal patients.[47]

Despite its perceived lowly status, numerically, asylum attendants dominated institutional nursing in England from *c.* 1860 until the end of the century.[48] It was a relatively attractive option compared to the rigours and uncertainty of seasonal employment, particularly for women. By 1861, 4,500 female attendants were reported to be working in licensed institutions for the insane.[49] By 1897, there were an estimated 20,000 male and female attendants employed in asylums 'countrywide'.[50] It might be argued that, initially, the best an asylum medical superintendent could hope for was a workforce that maintained relative sobriety, and which was physically and mentally strong enough to endure the long hours and hard labour. In spite of their numbers, the image of attendants as being of the lowest type was a persistent one for some historians.[51] Others, such as Digby, Smith and Wright, for example, have challenged this view, suggesting that this particular occupation was subject to local conditions and patterns of labour.[52] In some instances, asylums competed successfully in the local job market, although unfavourable comparisons have been drawn with other professions, especially for men.[53] Recruitment patterns were similar to that of general hospitals, and pay, notably from 1867 to 1881, was more than comparable to domestic service.[54] At Brookwood and Holloway, general male attendants could expect to be paid £25 to £35 per annum. Female attendants or nurses were paid £15 to £22, all with the additional benefit of inclusive board and lodging.[55] At Holloway, by 1900, a first-class, or senior, attendant could expect to be paid £40 to £45 per annum, a second-class attendant £33 to £39, and a third-class attendant £30 to £32.[56] The lady and gentlemen companions, despite their role being less physical, were paid at a slightly higher rate.

The nineteenth-century asylum attendant's work was arduous and potentially dangerous, not least because of the ever-present possibility of physical threats from the patients. The hours were long, and the attendants were as isolated as their patients and so, arguably, prone to institutionalization. The Commissioners in Lunacy were increasingly aware of the importance of recruiting and retaining hard-working and 'moral' attendants. Once employed, every aspect of their lives was subjected to close scrutiny. Their good personal behaviour was vital; it was seen to affect their ability to care for their patients but they were also expected to set a good example. From the late nineteenth century, regulation and the provision of training schemes were seen by most contemporaries as beneficial for individual workers and patients as well as for general asylum management.[57]

Recruitment

Brookwood, particularly during the early years, experienced a fairly rapid turnover in attendants, as those initially lured by the competitive wages and board often realized that they were unsuited to the rigours of asylum life. Some left either during or immediately after their first month's trial. Holloway's difficulties in retaining staff were often of a different nature. The introduction of formal training and subsequent qualifications encouraged some members of staff to seek promotional opportunities elsewhere, so that the sanatorium's investment was not repaid. Increased professionalization of attendants was not always advantageous; attempts to import similar training schemes for attendants in colonial

Australia, for example, were met with suspicion by the staff who felt it actually threatened their authority in the asylum.[58]

Although Brookwood and Holloway were of different sizes and catered for distinct classes of patients, both superintendents sought similar personal qualities and attributes in their attendants and nurses. Sobriety, honesty and high moral standards were crucial. As summarized by the *Handbook for the Instruction of Attendants on the Insane*, 'Attendants should be examples of propriety of conduct, order, personal neatness and perfect truthfulness'.[59] Whilst advertisements for staff in local and national newspapers and journals were usually brief, occasionally they specified additional requirements such as proficiency in sports or possessing musical ability. These social skills were seen as attractive by both sets of management, as they increased opportunities for recreational therapy.

Surviving staff records for Brookwood show that the male attendants came from a variety of occupational backgrounds. Information regarding their previous employment was not routinely recorded, but a few surviving application forms demonstrate that many male applicants had been in the armed forces, or had worked as skilled artisans.[60] A smaller proportion had worked in agriculture. Some applicants had previous experience as asylum attendants in either public or private institutions but this did not necessarily guarantee them the job, and this was found to be the case with other asylums, private or public.[61]

The preferred male applicants were relatively young and single. A military background was seen as advantageous as it demonstrated the ability to both administer and receive discipline. Recent military experience also increased the likelihood that the applicant had retained the level of health and fitness that was deemed so necessary for coping with asylum work. The suitability of these men was enhanced if they had participated in the regimental choir or band, as music was integral to asylum life both as therapy and entertainment. Sporting abilities were also viewed positively; it was an indication of healthy inclinations and the ability to engage the patients in physical activities. If an applicant possessed a former trade or practical skill, such as plumbing or carpentry, for example, this was also an asset. The new attendant would then have the potential to take on the additional responsibility of supervising a small patients' workshop which was medically therapeutic and contributed to the asylum's drive for self-sufficiency.[62]

One of several male skilled artisans who applied to join Brookwood's opening work force was the 27-year-old unemployed Joseph Carter from Cowley. Initially, Carter had trained as a plumber and painter, although later he joined the Fourth Dragoon Guards, Oxfordshire. In his application, he stressed his musical ability (he played several instruments including the trombone) and that he had been a member of a regimental choir. He also provided details of his previous experience of working with the insane, which he had gained from four years employment under the supervision of his father, who had been head attendant at Oxford's Littlemore Asylum.[63] Joseph initially was engaged as a hall porter at Brookwood, during which time he created a favourable impression and was duly promoted in 1868 to first-class attendant. This 'career path' was not unusual, in that several men and women joined the asylum staff as domestic servants before they were promoted to become attendants. This action would often be taken fairly quickly if was necessary to fill any sudden gaps created by departing attendants.

Regrettably, Joseph Carter's career as an attendant was rather short-lived. Excessive alcohol consumption or licentious behaviour was not tolerated by Brushfield, or indeed, by subsequent superintendents and senior doctors. After only one month in his new post, Carter was dismissed on the spot 'For improper conduct with a housemaid'. This was one Annie Taylor who had joined the asylum staff in January that year and who suffered the same fate.[64] Carter pursued his career in asylum employment, but seemingly rather unsuccessfully, as indicated by a letter to Brushfield a few years later from Octavious Sepson, superintendent of the City of London Lunatic Asylum at Stone, near Dartford. He asked if Brushfield knew a certain Joseph Carter:

> an Oxford man – a retired soldier, and a good musician; and if so, what were the circumstances under which he left you? He has been with me some time, and is now leaving under peculiar circumstances; it has only just come to my knowledge that he had been at Brookwood as he failed to mention the circumstance.[65]

Brushfield's response is unknown, but this episode indicates a level of collaboration between asylum superintendents regarding the difficulties of engaging suitable staff. It also shows that attendants would seek advancement or better conditions by applying to other asylums and hospitals for the insane.

Many female Brookwood attendants had previously been in domestic service. Asylum work was attractive to single women as board and lodging were provided in a similar way. There were several applications from domestic servants outside the local area, such as 36-year-old Sarah Frost, from Colchester. A single woman, Sarah was unemployed and homeless, as her services were no longer required in a 'situation' in Lincolnshire. Previously, she had worked as a governess, a housekeeper, and a shop assistant.[66] Sarah Farrington's age was unknown when she wrote in desperation to the asylum in August 1867. She described her unemployment as being the result of a severe family dispute that led to her being obliged to leave her job at Chester Asylum and take temporary lodgings nearby.[67] Although asylum employment was not easy, for some women it was definitely preferable to some other occupations. It cannot be said that the work of an asylum attendant was seen as a last resort, although there are not many surviving applications or correspondence to enlighten as to the primary motives for taking up such a position. Clearly conditions at Brookwood were, for some, preferable than those at other institutions and some attendants returned to Brookwood. On 6 March 1877, Eliza Rouse wrote to Brushfield from her employment at Fulham prison:

> Sir,
>   I beg to take the liberty of writing to ask if you have a vacancy as I am leaving here. I do not like the prison. I thought of speaking to you when I was down at the Ball but did not like to trusting you will favour me with an answer
>   I am Sir yours
>   Obediently Eliza Rouse

Brushfield wrote to her on 12 March telling her that he was willing to reinstate her as a second-class attendant.[68]

At Holloway, Rees Philipps and his successors also continually tried to attract, and retain, reliable and proficient male and female attendants. Unfortunately, fewer records have survived for this institution so less is known about the applicants. Wealthier patients often brought their own servants with them which occasionally caused difficulties amongst the residential staff as often these patients (and their servants) were unwilling to take orders from the sanatorium attendants and nurses whom they regarded as their social inferiors. Gentility was felt to be especially necessary when it came to caring for the sanatorium's female patients.[69] Rees Philipps, recognizing this, generally attempted to recruit higher calibre staff:

> On the ladies side, additional lady nurses, of good social position, have been engaged. Of the sympathetic kindliness, tact, and thoroughness with which some of the gentlewomen on the staff have carried out their duty to the lady patients, I cannot speak too highly.[70]

He paid tribute to all his female staff for their 'kindliness, tact, and thoroughness' which was very much valued.[71] In his opinion, educated and socially skilled employees displayed more appropriate behaviour and were more easily accepted by the middle-class patients. This was particularly important when it came to the sizeable proportion of non-certified patients, or voluntary boarders, who were seen as far more demanding and troublesome.

Discussing his male attendants in his 1896 annual report (by this time female attendants were usually referred to as nurses), Dr Rees Philipps placed a high premium on recruiting well-educated attendants who were also in robust physical health. He observed that the primacy of physical over scholastic aptitude was much debated amongst asylum superintendents. It was his firm opinion that the monotonous nature of asylum work naturally made attendants prone to mental and moral deterioration. He believed that this could be mitigated to some extent by employing attendants who were physically strong and actively engaged in some type of sporting activity. These attributes helped attendants survive the rigours of asylum work, but also, he argued, these qualities encouraged the patients to elevate their behaviour. Philipps firmly informed the General Committee in 1896:

> I will not again recommend the appointment of a male officer who has not some healthy athletic instincts. The good example which is set to patients by a medical officer, whose life is healthy and cleanly, and whose habits of work and play are keen and active, is of infinite value in the moral treatment of the insane.[72]

Some of the successful applications reflect the particular qualities that were sought by Rees Philipps. William Collis, age twenty-four, had been employed at Wellington College as a domestic servant, but he had also been a member of their volunteer fire brigade. Although not musical, he was a keen footballer and cricket player. He was engaged in 1897 for £25 per annum as his skills were seen as more important than his social class. Musical and sporting proficiency remained important criteria. William Clark, 21, had been an insurance agent. He also played football and cricket and was a competent cornet player who was employed for £30 per annum. Likewise, ex-soldier Albert Ellis, twenty-six, who rode and swam, and counted his previous trades as hot water fitter and general smith, was employed on the same salary in 1906.[73]

At both institutions, most male and female asylum attendants were young and single, and although marriage was the most frequent reason female employees resigned, the employment of male attendants and their wives was not uncommon.[74] Richard and Annie Williams joined Brookwood on 21 September 1868 as first- and second-class attendants respectively. Within a year, Annie was promoted to first-class attendant, and in June 1881, she and her husband were put in charge of Brookwood's new dairy farm. In addition to their salary, they received additional benefits that included an unfurnished apartment, with all their meals and laundry provided. This arrangement appeared to have suited them very well as they remained there until their retirement in May 1906.[75] It is possible that Brookwood was not averse to employing married couples as it provided a solution to the continued high turnover of female attendants. In 1886 this had caused the Commissioner in Lunacy to remark that only half of the current nurses had been employed for more than one year. This applied to less than a quarter of the male attendants.[76] It seems to have been the reverse at Holloway, possibly because its gentility made it more attractive to female employees. Following comments by the Commissioners in Lunacy, in 1899, the salaries of Holloway's male attendants were increased in an attempt to stem the loss of trained male attendants after their two-year qualification period.[77]

Given the close proximity of Brookwood to Holloway, it is not surprising that occasionally staff moved between these two establishments as well as to

other Surrey institutions. In his work on the Earlswood Asylum, David Wright
highlighted female attendants' migration from Brookwood, suggesting this was
prompted by the more favourable working conditions offered at Earlswood (a
voluntary asylum). The wages were the same, but the staff-to-patient ratio was
higher, which eased the physical burden.[78] However, female staff moved there
for promotional reasons, too; Julia Goodwin was engaged as a housekeeper at
Brookwood in December 1868 where she worked until April 1870 when she left
to take up the post of matron at Earlswood.[79]

Such movements were largely, but not exclusively, generated by single attendants and nurses, but married couples also sought fresh opportunities, and the
movement was by no means confined to a drain from Brookwood, as Wright
suggests. In 1899, Jacob Robertson was taken on as head attendant at Holloway
and given the additional duties of supervising the outdoor staff.[80] His wife was
employed as housekeeper. Less than one year later, the Robertsons left Holloway
for the larger and more austere Brookwood. On 11 February 1890, Jacob began his
duties as head male attendant on a salary of £180 per annum that was paid jointly
to Mr and Mrs Robertson, although the latter's role was unclear. The Robertsons
enjoyed a successful career at Brookwood. Jacob was made steward in November
1890, a post which he retained for nine years (until May 1899). By this time, their
joint earnings had risen to £300 with all board and lodgings provided.[81] One factor in their decision to move to Brookwood may have been the inadequate staff
accommodation at Holloway, which was frequently debated at Committee meetings. To address this, special cottages were eventually allocated to attract more
married attendants and other workers, but this did not happen until 1900.[82]

One of Brookwood's best known and longest serving employees was Robert
Lloyd, the head gardener who also designed the asylum's grounds.[83] This was not an
exclusive role; during his thirty-three years at Brookwood, where he remained until
his death in 1900, he and his wife acted as attendant and matron at their 'cottage',
where they cared for up to twelve patients at a time. After his death, his son, John
Godfrey Lloyd, also with his wife, continued to look after patients in their home. In
some respects, the care provided by the Lloyd family, albeit under the supervision of
the medical superintendent, was similar to that which occurred earlier in the nineteenth century when husband-and-wife teams were put in charge of insane patients,
as seen at both the York Retreat and at the sprawling Hanwell Public Asylum.[84]

Duties and Work

In keeping with other asylums, the working day for attendants at Brookwood
and Holloway often exceeded fourteen hours, and the week comprised six and a
half days.[85] Many common duties existed, although the class of patient did have
some bearing on the quality and structure of the attendant's day. For example,

Brookwood patients were much more likely to be given scheduled manual tasks to keep them employed.[86]

The varying ratio of staff to patients influenced the attendant's working regime and, as suggested by Melling and Forsyth, was indicative of the quality of life for staff and patients alike.[87] The situation at Exminster appears to have been especially dire, standing at 18.0 male patients to one (male) attendant in 1870, and 16.6 female patients to one (female) attendant.[88] At Brookwood, the more favourable ratio of staff to attendants was 10.5 male and 12.6 female patients per attendant. Additional night-time attendants were engaged and these ranged from five on the male side to seven on the female. For many years, a patient had assisted the night attendant in the infirmary ward, and while this was a common enough practice in workhouses, the Commissioners in Lunacy were critical, and it eventually ceased in 1889.[89]

By way of contrast, Holloway operated with a staff ratio of three patients to one attendant on both the male and female sides until *c.* 1890, when it became one to two. It appears to have remained at this level; in 1896 Rees Philipps reported that a total of 400 patients and boarders resided in the sanatorium (including the seaside branch) and that they were cared for by 160 attendants and nurses, or just over two patients to one member of staff.[90] This was private, almost individual care and, one may suppose, was some of the best that could be obtained without resorting to more expensive private institutions. It was also a better ratio than had been achieved by Rees Philipps at his previous private establishment, Wonford House in Devon.[91] The patient to staff ratio at Holloway was comparable to that found at The Retreat in York, where one attendant to 1.25 patients was recorded in 1900.[92]

These high ratios did not necessarily ensure the inmates' safety; attempted suicides and accidents were no fewer at Holloway than elsewhere and, unfortunately, the sanatorium was at the centre of some rather sensational and newsworthy incidents.[93] Rees Philipps was keenly aware of the problems associated with caring for the middle and upper classes, and controversially speculated whether the high staff-to-patient ratios actually contributed to the difficulties regarding their care, as it was personally intrusive. He believed that more staff did not necessarily mean that the patients were gainfully occupied or better cared for. He contrasted the situation at Holloway with his earlier years at other establishments, where only two attendants had cared 'admirably' for seventy patients:

> The huge staffing now-a-days employed is not an unmixed advantage for the patients. It is well known that occupation and work are valuable curative agents, and in the best managed asylums, in the old days, when staffs were smaller, more persistent efforts were necessarily made to occupy and employ the patients.[94]

However, the Commissioners in Lunacy strongly approved of this high ratio of attendants to patients at Holloway which they saw as essential given the layout of the sanatorium and its grounds, which made surveillance difficult. Although earlier difficulties concerning the sanatorium's design had delayed the opening, those issues had been addressed and the modifications had meant that the asylum met the legal requirements. Yet, as late as 1889, the Commissioners believed that that Rees Philipps still faced a difficult task in adapting the hospital 'to the requirements of lunatics'.[95]

The improvement and preservation of the patients' bodily health was a priority for all asylum attendants, and encompassed personal and environmental cleanliness, nourishing food, clothing, warmth, regular exercise and undisturbed sleep.[96] At Brookwood, the poor health of many new patients meant they required additional nursing and feeding in order to regain their bodily strength. This was time-consuming, and created additional pressure for the staff. Once stronger, the patients could become more difficult for the staff to control. Many workhouse patients were difficult or violent, and included large numbers of young single males who had a potential for disruption, self-harm and suicide. In his report for 1885, the superintendent observed that:

> The number of dangerous and suicidal patients in the wards have severely taxed the vigilance of the attendants, and have proved a source of much trouble and anxiety to the medical staff; and it is a matter for congratulation that the casualties have been few, and that, although several attempts at suicide were made, none were attended with fatal results.[97]

The incidents referred to included two attempted suicides, a female patient who choked to death, and a violent dispute between two patients that resulted in one receiving a broken rib.

Strict adherence to a daily regime in all asylums was essential for their smooth operation, and the doctor's instructions in all matters were strictly enforced. Routine was vital to maintain order and safety, but the 'regular hours' of the various activities were also seen as beneficial to bodily and mental health.[98] Each day, patients were awoken, bathed (or at least washed) and dressed, and their meals served. In the evening, this pattern was reversed and then day attendants were replaced by night nurses who kept careful watch, particularly with regard to any suicidal or epileptic inmates. During the day, patients were supervised whilst at meals, work, exercise and recreation. By necessity, the asylum day began and ended early, but every moment was strictly controlled and monitored. The attendants' daily work, which ranged from the banal to the dirty and downright dangerous, led many female employees to resign. In 1886, six months had been enough time to convince Nurse Jane Fleetwood that she was unlikely to fully settle at Brookwood, and, in the same year, Ella Miller resigned after her one month's probation period, as she disliked the work and was terrified of the patients. Other female members of staff were also fearful, such as the laundry woman who resigned after only three days, declaring herself nervous of the patients.[99]

The potential for patient unpredictability was ever-present and, with it, the threat of assaults from violent patients, both male and female. Reporting on Brookwood for 1885, the superintendent, Dr James Barton wrote:

> In January, a female patient threw a water-bottle at one of the charge nurses with such force that the bottle broke, and the nurse's face was much cut and disfigured, and she had a narrow escape of losing her eyesight. In April, a female patient, while at break-fast, threw a heavy delf [*sic*] cup at the senior charge nurse of F10, which struck her on the back of the head, producing concussion. This blow gave rise to grave mental symptoms, and the nurse was under medical treatment for a considerable time, but was eventually able to return to duty.[100]

He added that he, too, had been assaulted, by an ex-criminal who struck him forcefully in the face whilst on his ward visit.[101] Also at Brookwood, in 1893, a female patient, whilst in the throes of a maniacal frenzy, seriously attacked a nurse. During the course of the struggle, the patient suffered a fatal heart attack. The subsequent inquest exonerated the staff from all blame.[102] The same year, two other nurses were attacked by patients and, as a result, were reported as suf-fering from 'temporary disablement from concussion of the brain'.[103]

Similar to Brookwood, Holloway's management recognized that their rela-tively isolated location and consequent difficulties in accessing more 'urban pleasures' could make asylum work unattractive to young attendants. The super-intendent was convinced that a high staff turnover was financially damaging and so determined to establish a self-sufficient institution on all levels. Further, Rees Philipps observed that whilst the staff were generally satisfactory, they did not stay long; this was financially damaging and was partially attributed to the meagre accommodation that was provided for them at the sanatorium.[104] He urged the Committee to swiftly resolve the matter, believing that in doing so 'we shall probably find much greater contentment, and much better service, among both attendants and servants'.[105] At Brookwood, some female employees also complained about the relative isolation; in 1886, after only nine months' employment, Mary Ellen Ledwith, a night nurse, handed in her resignation 'because she finds the Country too lonely'.[106]

Discipline and Performance

The moral character of asylum attendants was an ongoing concern for both institutions and, as mentioned, every aspect of their behaviour, both inside and outside the workplace, was closely scrutinized. The demanding nature of the work necessitated alert, disciplined employees. Short shrift was accorded those members of staff found to be overindulging in alcohol, whether on duty or not. A beer allowance had been incorporated as one of the recognized 'perks' for asylum attendants for many years and this had remained the case at Brookwood until 1895.[107] In Superintendent George Thomson's view, beer noticeably worsened the conduct of attendants at Bristol Asylum (1885), and drunkenness was the most common disciplinary problem in all asylums, especially for male staff.[108] There are many recorded instances at both asylums of attendants and nurses being dismissed for drunkenness. James Atkins, a plumber attendant at Brookwood, was dismissed for neglecting his duties through intemperance. In December 1868, he had even taken a patient with him for company on a visit to a nearby public house.[109] George Richie, hired as dispenser in December 1877, did not last a month and was dismissed after being discovered 'in a stupor from drink or inhalation'.[110]

Detailed security guidance was issued to the attendants and nurses in respect of locks and keys, but also with regard to personal security and the monitoring of sharp instruments, tools and other items that could be used to self-harm or aid escape. If patients did escape, this could also lead to the prompt dismissal of attendants, as in the case of Samuel Ede, whose patient ran away in 1868.[111] Attendants were often held responsible for the recapture of their patients and were occasionally ordered to contribute towards the costs. Several occurrences such as this appeared in the Visitors' Minutes: 'George Davis a Patient having escaped through the neglect of W Richardson an attendant, a fine of 5 shillings is imposed on the said W Richardson.'[112]

Brookwood's first superintendent, Brushfield, frequently adopted a paternalistic role towards his attendants, particularly with regard to the welfare of the female employees, the majority of whom were single. In the case of Brookwood's female attendants, there was the additional problem of the close proximity of the army barracks at Pirbright that were seen to encourage 'immoral behaviour', unauthorized leave and staff shortages when female staff left to marry their soldiers.[113] Immorality was grounds for immediate dismissal if encountered within either asylum; second-class attendant James Cummings was dismissed after six months at Brookwood when it was discovered that he had written a series of indecent letters to a female attendant. The use of improper language on a ward was also inexcusable, and was the reason for the dismissal of Emma Elliot in 1879 after nearly fifteen months' service.[114]

The superintendent reported that changes in the attendants for 1886 at Brookwood had been rather too numerous: eight had left to be married, seven 'for a change' and a further three to 'better themselves'. Another three were dismissed for drunkenness, one for striking a patient and one for refusing to obey orders. One attendant had absconded and taken his uniform with him, so that a warrant was immediately issued for his arrest. Eventually he was apprehended at Southampton, brought before the Guildford Bench and sentenced to one month's hard labour. In spite of this, Dr Barton remained optimistic: 'The minor Staff, taken as a whole, have, I consider, performed their arduous duties with care, consideration and kindness'.[115]

Aside from the individual incidents which had to be investigated and recorded in the annual reports, the overall performance of the attendants is difficult to assess accurately, although usually the superintendents of Brookwood and Holloway talked favourably of their staff's diligence and hard work in caring for large numbers of patients. Circumstances in the asylums were often acknowledged as being particularly difficult, for example when building work was in progress or there was an outbreak of a contagious disease.

Maltreatment of patients by attendants was not tolerated at either institution, although less overt incidents such as rough handling, sly slaps or pushes, or withholding of food or privileges would have gone largely undetected. Occasionally, attendants lost their patience with their charges. If they were caught, or if strong complaints were received from the patients' relatives, action was taken. In 1889, a nurse was 'summarily dismissed' from Holloway by the superintendent for violence toward a female patient. A warrant was issued, and she duly appeared at Chertsey Police Court, but the magistrates dismissed the charge.[116] At Brookwood, Edward Freeman, a second-class attendant, only lasted five months before he was dismissed 17 September 1868 for striking a patient. For a similar offence, John Bedford was sacked on 3 January 1875 after fourteen months' service. Incidents such as these were not uncommon, particularly in the early years, when the records show that some attendants lost their positions as a result of rough handling or for using inappropriate language towards patients. Although such occurrences were more frequent amongst male employees, this was not exclusively the case.

Good attendants and nurses were at a premium, yet even the best made errors, often with serious consequences. The Tatford brothers, Albert and Joshia, began as first-class attendants at Brookwood in June 1867, and seem to have gone along uneventfully until August the following year. Whilst preparing to bathe a patient, Albert had left the filling bath unattended for a few minutes. It seems that he had run only the hot water tap so that when the patient climbed in, he sustained major burns. The patient died five days later and Albert was promptly dismissed for culpable negligence. The affair caused considerable embarrassment to Alfred's brother, Josiah, who felt it necessary to resign the following month.[117]

However, accidents did not necessarily impede an attendant's career, and the committees of both asylums were keenly aware of the pressures involved in working with the insane. In some instances, they were prepared to overlook quite serious errors in order to keep valued employees and maintain adequate staffing levels. Emily Vosey had been provided with a satisfactory, if rather uninspiring, reference from Dr Orange, superintendent of Broadmoor Criminal Asylum (also in Surrey), where she had worked as an assistant attendant for nearly a year before she arrived at Brookwood. She was quickly promoted to first-class attendant.[118] Two years later, in 1869, she accidentally administered a fatal dose of carbolic acid to a 20-year-old female hawker suffering from dementia.[119] It was agreed at the subsequent inquest held before one of Surrey's coroners that the attendant had mistaken the bottle of carbolic acid for 'House Medicine' (a laxative mixture of salts and senna), and she was duly exonerated of all blame. She continued to be employed at Brookwood until her marriage in August 1870.[120] Not all were treated so leniently, and less so as higher professional standards came to be expected; in 1890, Charge Nurse Frances Abram was dismissed for gross negligence, despite her previous six years of unblemished employment, after she had administered the incorrect medicine to a patient.[121]

At Brookwood, there were several incidents which suggested possible staff negligence, and there were also inconsistencies in applying standards and administering punishment. Good character or favouritism may have contributed to the decisions made by the management of either establishment. Whilst, to some extent, the relative paucity of surviving records precludes a fuller comparison, Brookwood, being a public institution, was more accountable and so any staff shortcomings were more likely to be exposed. However, one area that invoked full investigative proceedings and consideration of possible neglect was that of suicide within the asylum. This was believed to be preventable, primarily by way of surveillance, the success of which rested on the ability and diligence of the attendants. There were completed suicide attempts in both institutions, but, perhaps surprisingly, given the staff ratios, more occurred at Holloway. In all cases, the attendant's culpability was unproven and their institutions were largely exonerated from blame.[122] This would suggest that, certainly from the 1870s, the time of the first suicide at Brookwood, asylum staff were diligent overall in the execution of their duties.

Although most nursing errors were not fatal, as the nineteenth century drew to a close, higher standards were increasingly expected of asylum attendants as part of the attempt to secure professional recognition. Prior to organized formal training, some superintendents took the initiative and arranged elementary talks for their staff on various aspects of nursing the insane. In 1885, the Medico-Psychological Association prepared the first edition of its *Handbook for the Instruction of Attendants on the Insane*, although most asylums had issued their own sets of instructions and rules for all levels of medical staff.[123] As Peter Nolan has pointed out, the publication of the *Handbook* was important, as it attempted to give the attendant's work some degree of scientific credibility and establish uniformity. At the same time, it conveyed the value of study, as those attendants who wished to advance had to be able to understand and quote from it.[124]

Holloway's Rees Philipps was an active member of the Asylum Workers Association (AWA) that was formed under the auspices of the Medico-Psychological
Association in 1895.[125] The AWA sought to promote the professionalization of
asylum staff, and improve the status of attendants and nurses, then estimated to
be 20,000 in number countrywide. The Association also aimed to gain the support of those interested in institutional work, as well as establishing a nursing
home for retired asylum workers.[126] In the early years, however, the AWA was
seen as paternalistic with its uplifting speeches, but attendants did not even go
to, let alone speak at, annual meetings. The first edition of their journal, *Asylum
News*, was published in 1897 (when the AWA had 2,000 members) and it argued
that the professional recognition of asylum workers would ultimately benefit
the patients. The organization was not, however, devoted solely to nurses and
attendants but also included the asylum doctors, laying it open to accusations
of primarily protecting management's power although seeming to advance the
interests of asylum employees.[127]

The training and professionalization of asylum attendants and nurses was
increasingly debated within the medical journals from the 1890s, but the advantages of specialized training and subsequent recognition were not agreed upon
by all. Some members of the Royal British Nurses Association publicly opposed
the registration of asylum attendants.[128] However, the Medical-Psychological
Association persisted with their scheme for formal instruction and examinations. To combat any accusations regarding lack of training, it was proposed
that asylum nurses and attendants serve their professional apprenticeship of two
years' duration in a hospital for the insane that was over forty beds in size. This
would include studying for a Certificate of the Medico-Psychological Association for nursing proficiency in this specialized field. In addition, nurses would
receive 'a certificate of moral character' where it was deemed to be appropriate.
This would encourage upright and sober personal behaviour on the part of the
attendants and nurses.[129] It was hoped that such training would inspire public confidence in their proficiency, a point that was eventually accepted by the
Council of the Royal British Nurses Association, who finally agreed to accept
the registration of asylum nurses and attendants, suitably trained and qualified,
but in a separate section of their Register.[130]

Holloway's management were enthusiastic about training their staff, and by
1895, thirty-three attendants and forty-one nurses had passed the Medico-Psychological Association's examination.[131] Each year the numbers increased. Arguably,
the prestige of asylum nursing rose and, given the luxurious surroundings and its
high staff-to-patient ratio, Holloway was an attractive location for training. One
female correspondent to the *Asylum News* who enquired as to where she could
obtain asylum training in an environment 'where nurses are refined and well-cared
for' was advised to write to Dr Rees Philipps at Holloway Sanatorium.[132]

This professionalization, however, caused some unexpected difficulties. Rees Philipps lamented that, once attendants and nurses had passed the rudimentary exams of the Medico-Psychological Association, some thought themselves fully qualified and quickly left in search of better paid positions felt to value their particular skills. To combat this, in 1901, the sanatorium established a new scheme, whereby silver medals were awarded to attendants and nurses who served over five years in addition to having gained a certificate of the Medico-Psychological Association in mental nursing.[133] Seventeen nurses and attendants were initially rewarded with medals in that year, although some Holloway nurses and attendants continued to seek prestigious positions elsewhere. During 1889, it was reported that one nurse left to become matron of the York Lunatic Hospital, and, somewhat more exotically, the deputy head attendant and his wife 'have been engaged at a handsome salary to undertake the organising of a public asylum for the Republic of Costa Rica.'[134] The same year saw Head Attendant Mr P. McLean leave to go into business; he was succeeded by Mr W. Kyles, 'who gave great satisfaction' during his short appointment, although he was clearly an ambitious man as he soon resigned to become general manager and private secretary to the Marquis of Breadalbane.[135]

Other Asylum Staff

The surviving records do not allow for a detailed consideration of the many other non-medical staff who were essential to the orderly running of these institutions. As identified, domestic servants were often promoted to the role of attendant, although even attendants incorporated some domestic tasks into their daily routine. There was a plethora of skilled and unskilled workers who assisted the asylum function and, in the case of Holloway, the numbers were inflated periodically by the arrival of some patients bringing their personal servants.

At Holloway Sanatorium, there were other members of staff engaged who were neither strictly medical, nor did they fall into the category of domestics. These were the lady and gentleman companions, employed by the medical superintendent to live amongst the patients in an effort to restore behavioural and social normality.[136] They participated in all aspects of the patients' daily lives, and were especially useful when the sanatorium's moral treatment included the introduction of social events, or alterations to routines. For example, in 1888, a table d'hôte dinner, followed by tea and music, was established for those patients who were well enough. This was presided over by the assistant medical officers who were assisted by the companions.[137] They were seen as an important addition to sanatorium life, and in his first annual report, Rees Philipps enthusiastically informed the Committee that almost immediately after opening, two male and female 'companions' had been engaged to live amongst the patients, 'and are of the greatest use in promoting occupation and amusement'.[138] By 1888, the number of lady companions had increased to seven and male companions to three. 'Most of these subordinate officials possess musical or artistic tastes, which are of advantage in promoting the comfort of the patients and borders.'[139] Louisa Fowle joined the sanatorium staff in 1894, accompanied by glowing references: 'She is a Lady by birth and by education'.[140] The 35-year-old spinster was the daughter of a Bridgewater clergyman, whom she had assisted with the daily running of his parish. She was accomplished in drawing, dancing and needlework, spoke French fluently, played tennis and was reputedly a good organist and pianist. She was employed on a salary of £30 per annum, once it was established that she would also become the sanatorium's organist and train their choir. She remained at Holloway until 1928.[141]

The post of chaplain was important for both asylums, as spiritual guidance was seen as necessary for both staff and patients, and a good clergyman ensured a well-attended asylum chapel, which pleased the Commissioners in Lunacy. Brookwood had employed its own chaplain from July 1867, and John Gillington remained in office until September 1884. He was paid a somewhat higher salary than his Holloway counterpart; £200 rising to £250 per annum, although accommodation was not provided for him until 1873.[142]

Holloway was originally visited by the local vicar, the Reverend Eales, but Rees Philipps found the *ad hoc* arrangement unsatisfactory and urged the General Committee to engage their own residential clergyman. He advised them that:

> To satisfactorily fill such a post the Chaplain must be a man of broad and liberal views, of some musical ability, genial in manner, and earnest in his work, one who can gain the confidence and respect of patients and staff.[143]

Eventually, Reverend Eales retired to make room for a permanent chaplain, the Reverend T. W. Hutchison, who was chosen from sixty-one applications, on a salary of £150 per year with a house provided.[144] He began his occasional duties in June 1888, moved into the asylum in December and was very popular: 'For several weeks Mr Hutchinson resided in the Hospital as a guest, and gave much satisfaction to the patients by the hearty way in which he joined in the general routine and the amusements of the House.'[145]

Conclusion

At Brookwood Asylum and Holloway Sanatorium, good management practices became increasingly important. There were areas of mutual concern, as both institutions struggled to provide a good level of care whilst negotiating future admissions and ensuring that there was sufficient capacity and staff to maintain good safety levels. Despite the fact that they primarily served different classes of patients, the first medical superintendents' long periods of office provided stability, continuity and strong leadership. Both superintendents sought to care for their patients and staff, despite financial constraints and complex issues of accountability. These were more pressing at Brookwood than at Holloway where Rees Philipps could explore new treatments more freely, engage in staff education at an earlier stage, and employ more varied types of staff, particularly female doctors and lady and gentleman companions.

For many years, both institutions endured the inconveniences of ongoing building work in an attempt to meet the increasing demand for places, as well as provide additional staff facilities. Superintendents struggled to keep therapeutic objectives to the fore, whilst beset by bureaucratic demands, increased form filling and recordkeeping. Having efficient and professional medical officers to whom routine tasks could be delegated, as well as reliable attendants and nurses to care for patients in the wards, were paramount in the successful running of these two asylums. As the patient population increased, so too did the need for extra attendants, and considerable care was taken to recruit suitable men and women from a variety of backgrounds. In most cases, transgression of the rules by attendants was dealt with promptly and strictly but, as we have seen, there were some inconsistencies where leniency and occasional exoneration of blame were exhibited. This may have been evoked by recognition of the difficulties and challenges of the job, as well as the inconsistent and variable nature of the patients whom they cared for.

Expectations of staff efficiency rose as knowledge increased and formal training was introduced to the advantage of patients and staff alike. Asylum attendants received benefits and opportunities and a relative degree of social and professional advancement. For working women, in particular, asylum employment offered unusual security and opportunities for independence.[146] The evidence here highlights that several married couples also benefited and took advantage of a double income accompanied by additional benefits.

Increased professionalization was not always beneficial for asylum management and it has been shown that attendants – single or married, with increased skills and confidence – often sought promotion and better conditions elsewhere. Hence, there were additional difficulties in retaining newly qualified staff. The employment of genteel companions at Holloway adds an interesting dimension to our understanding of asylum staff and hierarchy. They introduced an intermediate layer of employment to the sanatorium, where social status as much as occupational skills were important selection criteria. With their high staff-to-patient ratios Holloway could offer relative patient freedom in comparison to the less advantageously staffed Brookwood with its vigilant but more regimented care. The two staffing regimes had contrasting downsides in patient care, with more accidents and cases of negligence at Brookwood but relatively more suicides at Holloway.[147]

Whilst one asylum dealt with huge numbers of poor patients, and the other provided care for a smaller number of predominantly middle-class patients, the medical staff of both institutions sought similar outcomes: a return to normalization as designated by their patient's social status, assisted by engaging the best attendants and nurses that they could find. As role models, and in order to achieve this, all aspects of the attendants' lives were subjected to intense scrutiny and their behaviour regulated and monitored. In some respects, despite having greater freedom of choice, attendants' daily lives bore a strong resemblance to that of their patients and they could even become institutionalized, as suggested by the many years' service given by several members of staff.

3 ORIGINS AND JOURNEYS: THE PATIENTS AT BROOKWOOD ASYLUM AND HOLLOWAY SANATORIUM

Introduction

Although the two institutions were designed to care for different classes of patients, it is too simplistic to label Holloway Sanatorium a middle-class haven and Brookwood Asylum a stringent Poor Law asylum. This chapter examines the origins of the two patient populations and, in particular, provides an overview of the patients' journeys to institutional care, as well as their physical and mental condition on arrival.[1] These factors had implications for the medical outcomes of both male and female patients, and thus the 'success' of both establishments in caring for and treating their patients.

The patients did not simply suffer from mental disorders; Brookwood admitted many patients who were in a poor physical condition that often was the result of poverty, intensified by either long-term or seasonal unemployment. At both institutions, patients arrived with evidence of having been mistreated or neglected by their carers. Some patients were also undernourished and sometimes suffered from a range of additional illnesses at varying stages of severity. Yet others presented with a range of physical disabilities such as blindness or deafness which could prohibit an accurate diagnosis. These patients all required differing levels of care but it was the epileptic, dangerous and suicidal patients that provoked the most medical concern as these conditions could result in premature deaths in the asylum. Additional medical observations were implemented, such as a twenty-four hour watch or a suicide caution being issued for the actively suicidal.[2] Such is the importance of this particular group of patients that they are the subject of a dedicated chapter (see below, pp. 145–67). In addition, there were criminal patients incarcerated at Brookwood, while Holloway was obliged to admit Chancery lunatics.[3]

Pregnant or lactating women required additional nursing and care; babies born in the asylum (more often in Brookwood) were removed soon after birth, not least because both asylums were intended for adult lunatics. But, at a time when children's specialized care for mental disorders was only emerging, Brookwood found itself dealing with the regular admission of small numbers of children. These children had a very definite impact on the asylum environment; their presence strained resources and their vulnerability was a concern for the staff, especially as children as young as four were being taken into custody. They required close supervision and often needed protection from some of the more aggressive adult patients with whom they were incarcerated. By way of contrast, no children under the age of fifteen were cared for at Holloway during the time studied.

The Route into the Asylums

Large county asylums such as Brookwood were primarily intended to serve the insane poor, but the reality was more nuanced. In their detailed study of mental healthcare provision in Devon, Melling and Forsythe observed that the 'classical pauper' lunatic associated with the workhouse was not necessarily the typical nineteenth-century county asylum inmate.[4] David Wright's work on Buckinghamshire County Asylum also addressed the issue of what constituted a 'pauper lunatic'. He broadly endorsed an earlier definition by Peter McCandless that, within this context, the term 'pauper' was applied to those patients who did not contribute financially to the cost of their asylum treatment, as opposed to those who were destitute and in receipt of Poor Law relief.[5] This definition applies to the Brookwood patients, none of whom paid fees whatever their social status or financial position; unlike some other county asylums, Brookwood did not take any private patients. An overview of the patients' occupations (see below) indicates that, while most would have had severely limited financial resources, a significant number of patients originated from a skilled working-class background and that some were even of the professional classes.

Brookwood patients' origins contrast with those asylums which served a more rural populace; for example, Peter Bartlett's work on Leicestershire County Asylum shows that, in the 1860s, 60 per cent of inmates came to the asylum directly from their household and a further 20 per cent were first taken to the workhouse by their families before being sent on to the county asylum by the Guardians.[6] At Stone Asylum, in predominantly rural Buckinghamshire, workhouse admissions accounted for just under a quarter of all asylum admissions.[7] During the early nineteenth century, at the Devon County Asylum (which also cared for a largely rural population) the majority of new patients had been in employment and had not been previously destitute; most came from the local labouring, handicraft and service industries. Gradually, increased numbers of both sexes with no stated occupation were admitted, with approximately 36 per cent having been workhouse residents prior to their removal. To some extent, this has been attributed to the spread of industrialization to the county which impacted upon local employment and social trends which in turn led to varied and uneven developments in urban and rural class relationships.[8]

The majority of patients who arrived at Brookwood had previously been resident in the workhouse, another asylum or their home. As might be expected, initially a sizeable proportion were transferred from other institutions, such as the first county asylum at Wandsworth or from other public and private asylums that had been temporarily holding Surrey's insane whilst Brookwood was being constructed. In the first year after opening, the urban workhouses took the opportunity to hastily rid themselves of a great many of their more difficult lunatics. The pattern emerged of nearly equal numbers of new inmates coming to Brookwood from the workhouses (42 per cent in 1871 for example) as from their homes (45 per cent) and this remained a consistent picture until 1890.[9] By 1897 when more Brookwood patients originated from the rural areas of the county, a very slight decrease in the numbers of workhouse patients is perceptible, but, by 1900, 44 per cent came directly from home whilst workhouses accounted for 46 per cent of patients.[10] Overall, more women than men were transported from their homes but of those who came from the workhouses, there were roughly equal numbers of men and women.[11]

The workhouse environment facilitated individual surveillance, and an inmate's behaviour potentially alerted staff to the necessity of moving them to a more specialized and secure environment.[12] The badly behaved and difficult lunatic patients who disrupted the workhouse routine and strained resources were quickly identified and an application for their transferral made as soon as it became feasible. Many younger men fell into this category which is especially reflected in Brookwood's early admissions. However, women could also cause difficulties and, in this, the workhouse distaste for fractious patients was consistent. Jessie C., a 53-year-old widowed needlewoman diagnosed with mania, was brought to Brookwood from the workhouse in April 1900. Her accompanying medical certificate stated: 'She is beyond the control of the workhouse. She is suffering from delusions of identity and has hallucinations of sight and of hearing.' She was reported to have been talkative, excited, used bad language and caused general disruption in that 'She wanders about and will not obey our regulations.'[13] Workhouses could also be expressly used as a temporary holding area pending a patient's removal to the asylum, as seen in the policy decisions that were made in Leicester in 1846.[14] At Brookwood, the initial volume of applications from urban Surrey workhouses threatened to overwhelm the asylum, so within weeks of opening, the Committee of Visitors were obliged to restrict eight metropolitan unions to a collective total of 280 patients, with the highest allocation (36 per cent) awarded to the large Lambeth Union. By 15 October 1867, just five unions – Bermondsey, Lambeth, Newington, St George's Southwark, and St Saviour's – accounted for 34 per cent of the new patient intake to Brookwood.[15]

Surrey's rural workhouses accounted for an insignificant number of insane inmates admitted to Brookwood prior to 1890 which reflected the density of the county's population in the urban areas south of the Thames. But there were other factors, such as the reluctance of some to rid themselves of their insane inmates so easily. One such example was Guildford Workhouse; the Guardians highlighted the advantages of the care that they offered to the harmless lunatics of the local area, especially the easy access for family and friends. Determined to retain their inmates and provide long-term care, modifications were made to the workhouse accommodation in accordance with the legal and medical requirements.[16] In a similar vein, the City of London Union had actively promoted the many advantages and the high standard of care available for the lunatics within their workhouse, but they eventually were unable to prevent a sizeable majority being transferred to specialized accommodation in Kent.[17]

The Brookwood management frequently drew attention to the poor condition of some new patients, particularly, but not always, those who originated from workhouses. The main concern was medical, in that their general state of debility rendered most available treatments largely ineffective. Previous lack of care and attention, malnourishment and underlying chronic illnesses all adversely affected the possibility of patient recovery, which ultimately damaged the asylum's reputation. Some patients arrived at Brookwood under variable degrees of restraint which caused distress and sometimes resulted in bruises and fractures that exacerbated their already weakened condition. When workhouse patients arrived, their clothing was usually removed and burnt prior to their being bathed and receiving any medical attention. One year, the superintendent identified for the Committee five of the 'most unsatisfactory' admissions, four of which were women, who had been transferred to Brookwood from workhouses:

> Jane M., aged 27, received in a state of great exhaustion from a metropolitan workhouse. When brought her wrists were fastened together by handcuffs, and secured to a waistband; her ankles were also bound together. Both wrists and ankles much bruised by restraining apparatus, many bruises (some of a large size) on various parts of her body.
> Ann W., aged 22, brought from a metropolitan workhouse. A case of puerperal mania, and far advanced in phthisis; died within three weeks.
> 'Elizabeth D. B., aged 43, brought in a cab 14 miles from a country workhouse; admitted in a dying condition, and restrained by a sleeve jacket; died 7½ hours afterwards.
> Maria D., aged 81, a case of ordinary senile dementia, brought on October 25th from a metropolitan workhouse, in an apparently dying condition, and for a long time was in a state of much danger. Remains in the infirmary ward, and gives no trouble.[18]

Families chose the county asylum as a suitable place for difficult, although arguably not always insane, relatives for a variety of reasons. Some felt unable to cope with the wide range of behaviours demonstrated by an insane family member, or they feared being unable to keep them safe, both from harming themselves or others. David Wright has argued that, in the public asylum, families were critical of the confinement process, and that endeavouring to have their trouble-some relatives incarcerated was a calculated strategy adopted in response to the stresses induced by industrialization.

Many of the personal concerns and worries of the families of Brookwood's patients were not so dissimilar to those who took their relatives to be cared for at Holloway Sanatorium. In either case not all motivation can be presumed to be altruistic, nor was it viewed as such by the medical staff. At Brookwood, for example, Brushfield expressed his conviction in 1871 that many of his patients, particularly the elderly, had been sent to the asylum by their family and friends, 'for the mere purpose of getting them out of the way'. Such action was, in his view, indicative of an intrinsic lack of compassion amongst families and commu-nities, but, just as importantly, he believed that it was also medically damaging; these patients occupied valuable places that could be better filled by more medi-cally deserving cases.[19] The superintendent also viewed increased urbanization as a factor in dispatching harmless – but annoying – insane relatives to institu-tions. But overall, the true extent of family collusion in the committal process is difficult to unveil, although as shown, the evidence they provided was used in certifying both public and private patients.

Patients who were brought from home by relatives or friends were not always guaranteed to be in a better mental or physical condition than those transferred from workhouses or other institutions. Fear, or lack of understanding, could result in some families handling their relatives too roughly; for example, in 1869, one newly arrived male patient especially warranted the superintendent's concern:

> George B., aged 66, brought from his own home. The whole of his left arm greatly swollen and bruised, and on examination a comminuted fracture into the elbow joint was detected. This injury of more than a week's standing, had remained unnoticed, and without treatment up to the day of his admission. Had been four times an inmate of other Asylums.[20]

But for most families whose relatives and friends were admitted to Brookwood, the incarceration process was usually traumatic, just as it was for some of the middle classes who chose Holloway for their loved ones. Their concerns, wor-ries and feelings of helplessness are evident in the contents of some of their correspondence to the Brookwood authorities. Often, their chief concern was the discharge of their relatives from the asylum; usually, this was something that they actively sought, but not always, as will be seen later in this chapter.

Caroline W. was admitted 27 August 1867 in a maniacal state, and suffering from a breast infection. The medical opinion was that she might have been suf-fering from puerperal insanity following the recent birth of her first child. Her husband, a labourer from Bermondsey Street, Southwark, wrote a concerned letter to the Superintendent:

> Dear Sir, I was verrey sorrey to hear that my wife Caroline Walsh was taken so Bad I hope it will not be for long Please God her Babey is getting on as well as can be expectted with the mother I hope yo [you] will be kind and to let me know when she is likely to be fit for home
>> Please do remember me to my wife and give my kind love to her.
>> I remain yours truley, Thomas Walsh.[21]

Her father also wrote in to the authorities enquiring after his daughter's health and her possible release date. Fortunately for her family, who would have been unable to make the journey, Caroline was only an inmate for just over four months, endorsing the original view that this was a short-lived acute condition, such as puerperal insanity, arguably one of the most easily identifiable psychiatric conditions in the nineteenth century.[22] Caroline was discharged 'Recovered' on the 9 January 1868; the doctor recorded in her case notes that: 'She is rather weak and silly, but this, it has been ascertained, she has always been.'[23] Many surviving letters contained simple requests for information regarding the physical and mental well-being of their relatives or asked when they could visit; sometimes they petitioned for their release. Often families would do their best to emphasize their ability to provide adequate care for their relatives in their attempt to have them discharged as early as possible. The loving parents of Fanny H. from Rotherhithe, admitted to Brookwood in December 1875, were aware of their daughter's 'excitable' nature, but after seventeen months' incarceration they began the process to have her returned to their care, writing to the superintendent on 8 May 1877:

> Dear Sir,
>> In reply to your respecting my daughter Fanny H I must tell you she was always very excited from a child but she never attempted to do any thing rash, she has written twice to me and in her letters she says she has implored Dr Barton to let her come home and I think Sir she will never be any better while she remains in the Asylum being in very good health I think Sir I may venture to have her home again if you permit Her father Sister likewise myself will be answerable for her, Sir I have a great wish to have her home if her father came on Friday and brought her clothes would you allow him to fetch her or must Mr White come or must they both come would you kindly write back and let me know. I am not afraid Sir she will do any harm I have such a great wish to have her home with me again. [24]

The reply from the superintendent advised the parents that they could make a personal application to the visiting magistrates at the asylum on Friday 18 May; however it was not until 15 March 1878 that Fanny was finally discharged to the custody of her parents as 'not improved'.[25]

Yet other families expressed their fears or reluctance to receive a relative back into the fold. Kate W. wrote in consternation to Brushfield regarding the possible discharge of her father Henry who had been admitted in December 1877 suffering from melancholia. The 56-year-old surgeon had spent twelve days in Lambeth Infirmary before being moved to Brookwood where he was admitted in a delusional and rambling condition. This was the third attack he had suffered as a result of 'overstudy and drink'.[26] Henry, given his stated occupation, was not working class but earning a living as a surgeon in the nineteenth century could be precarious. His intemperance may have lost him patients (and therefore income), so that he may have been unable to pay for private treatment.[27] Alternatively, his immediate relatives may not have been willing or able to do so, as suggested by his daughter's letter.

As Alannah Tompkins has pointed out, the numbers of medical practitioners admitted to asylums were relatively small but similarly to other professional men in general, medical practitioners, whatever their area of specialization, were vulnerable to nervous exhaustion, stress, nervous breakdown and insanity.[28] Henry's diagnosis conforms to an extent. His short stay at Brookwood was largely unremarkable; his sleeplessness was administered to as required and on one occasion he was recorded as being melancholy and suicidal. Seemingly sufficiently lucid, he wrote to his daughter about what he hoped would be his forthcoming discharge, provoking this frantic letter addressed to Dr Brushfield on 28 March 1878:

Sir,
I must apologise for such a hurried untidy letter as I wrote to you yesterday, but I was so anxious not to lose any time before writing for fear I should be too late. I must repeat my urgent request that you should keep him or transfer him (to where they would keep him) please do. Papa states in his letter that, as his transfer is delayed, it is thought that he had better be discharged from Brookwood which he hopes will be Friday week. Is this true? If so, please do alter your decision for I do not know what will become of him. Will you forgive & have patience with me if I intrude my private affairs upon you, that you may see clearly, how matters stand.

My salary is £5.8s.4d. per calendar month at 25s. per week. If papa came, my rent which is now ⅞ for two rooms must be increased, I know at least to 10/– even if Mrs Pipe would allow me to stay then which I do not think. I cannot get cheaper about here.

Board for two cannot be less than 10/ just double what I now allow myself
Washing for two with bed & table linen ⅜
Light ⅙ per week

This amounts to 10s + 10 + 3.6 + 1.6 = £1.5 just the amount of my salary & allows nothing for any little extras, clothing travelling expense or even such tiny things as paper & ink or needles & cottons (As to his getting up a Practice & so it only being for a few days! as he states, I am positive he will not be able to do that, at least in his present condition; old patients know his failing too well new, he has neither strength of mind or energy, at present, to obtain. You cannot think Sir, what pain it gives me to say all this of my only Parent who is all to me now I have lost Mama but I think it is my duty under existing circumstances)

From the above, can I do as Papa wants me? Friends will not help, I tried some last night & they wish me to clearly understand they will do nothing for him or help me. His own relations are too poor to support themselves properly.

What can I do? It seems so hard to shut up a man of his age, talent & capabilities; but judging from what I last saw of him, I do not think he is at all fit to be set free, to act for himself & be entirely without control or fear of anyone. Do you think so. – If not troubling you too much, I hope to come down next Saturday to speak to you about the case.

Please excuse my great rudeness in writing to you as I have done but I felt obliged or you would not have known exactly about things.[29]

This letter, apparently the second one Kate had written to the superintendent (the first has not survived), is unusual in the amount of detail it contains as well as the clarity about the domestic and financial situation of a patient's family. Henry's daughter wrote in an educated hand and clearly set out her expenses, giving a fascinating picture of how a respectable but relatively poor single woman was living in Hackney at that time.[30]

It is not known how Brushfield responded to her appeal, but not long after her letter, her father was discharged as 'Improved'. He was sent to Bethnal House Asylum on 11 April 1878, possibly sponsored by a medical charity, but it is more likely that he was being held there prior to his transfer to Leavesden Pauper Asylum in Hertfordshire once a place became available.[31] This was unusual for a surgeon; as Tompkins has suggested, when it came to medical practitioners, they and their families preferred to apply for admission to private licensed houses (presumably they were thought to be more discreet) over the charitable hospitals or Poor Law asylums.[32]

The poor physical and mental condition of many patients who were transferred to Brookwood from other asylums led them to be usually labelled as incurable. Fortunately, other than immediately after opening and later with the realignment of the county borders, most years these transfers only accounted for around 5 per cent of the new inmates. But even so, most years they adversely affected Brookwood's recovery rates. The asylum also consistently contained a small number of criminal lunatics who were transferred from the nearby criminal asylum, Broadmoor, as well as from regular Surrey prisons such as Woking Convict Prison, Wandsworth House of Correction and Horsemonger Lane Gaol in Southwark.[33] These men and women had been convicted for a wide range of offences, from infanticide to larceny to horse theft. Some prisoners were moved to Brookwood after the expiration of their sentence, others during their prison term if they were judged by the authorities to have become insane and difficult to manage during their imprisonment.[34] On 15 August 1864, Rosa Mc.

was charged at the Central Criminal Court with 'wounding with intent to do grievous bodily harm' and sentenced to seven years' penal servitude. During her prison term, her behaviour was observed to have deteriorated and she was transferred to Brookwood on 28 August 1871, aged thirty-two. By 9 November, her maniacal and aggressive behaviour had escalated alarmingly, to the extent that she was relocated to Broadmoor where she served out the remainder of her sentence.[35] Once this was completed, she was examined and found to be still insane and so was once more returned to Brookwood where she continued throughout her incarceration to be delusional, violent and abusive to staff and patients.[36]

The route to institutional care for most Holloway patients differed considerably from those sent to Brookwood and most came directly from their own homes. The remainder were transferred from other, mainly private, institutions, although a very small number came from county asylums where management policy had allowed small numbers of private patients who were a source of additional income. Most admissions had been certified, but not always; a sizeable number were 'voluntary boarders' or uncertified patients, although their status could alter during their stay.

The voluntary patients' admission process, which was very much favoured by Holloway authorities, was an important factor in determining some principles of incarceration in the nineteenth century, particularly for the middle classes. Increasingly, the Commissioners in Lunacy voiced their concern regarding the use of this process at Holloway, believing it to be open to abuse or mismanagement. Holloway's management was not unique in favouring the admission of voluntary boarders, or as one contemporary advocate called them, the 'semi-sane'.[37] Admitting voluntary boarders to Holloway accorded with middle-class sensibilities, and, whilst it could facilitate certification if that was required, their early admission could potentially avoid that next step by offering timely intervention in a calm and benign environment. A further advantage was that 'voluntary patients know they are free agents, and have confidence that all will be done that can be to restore them to health'.[38] For many it was an attractive option, and, as Melling has pointed out, familial sensitivity helped sustain the pre-1890 certification system for private patients that required only the authority of two doctors and a relative – without the support of a magistrate or Poor Law authority – as was needed for all admissions to the public asylum.[39]

Due to the close proximity of Holloway Sanatorium to the metropolis, many patients originated from the better areas of London, as well as from other predominantly southern towns and cities, such as Brighton, Bristol, Bournemouth, Canterbury and Cheltenham. A few came from abroad, often from the colonies (including India and Australia), but also from other countries, including Belgium, Egypt and France. The men were usually British subjects who had lived overseas, perhaps while employed in the diplomatic or armed services, and the women were their wives and relatives.

Several cases of both certified and voluntary patients were admitted to Holloway on variable scales of charitable assistance, and some patients were routinely admitted *gratis*. But the grandeur and beauty of this institution also made it very appealing to the upper echelons of society. The management was soon obliged to accept several high fee-paying cases so as to meet financial needs. This change in policy subtly altered the charitable ethos of the sanatorium, similar to The Retreat in York where the growing number of non-Quaker admissions had become increasingly dominated by upper-class patients from the north of England.[40] Amongst both certified and voluntary high fee-paying patients at Holloway, there were a small number of Chancery lunatics (or Lunatics by Inquisition) who were regularly scrutinized by committees and other interested parties.[41] Holloway also took in and boarded some poor lunatics via the After-Care Association; these were no longer 'patients' as such, but discharged men and women from other institutions who were seen to still require some continued form of care and assistance.[42] These two groups arguably represented opposing ends of the social scale, neither of which were representative of the middle-class patients for whom Holloway Sanatorium had originally been intended. No patients were transferred to Holloway directly from any workhouse, but occasionally criminally insane inmates of the middle classes were admitted. John W. was transferred to the sanatorium on 6 September 1887 from Broadmoor Criminal Asylum where he had been confined since 11 October 1881. He had been found guilty of 'feloniously wounding with intent to murder' a sixteen-year-old female servant from his Peckham lodgings. Allegedly instructed by 'voices', and following a heavy day's drinking in Margate, he had tried to cut her throat with a razor, after which he retreated to his room where he attempted suicide by the same method. During his trial it was disclosed that he had previously spent a year at Peckham House whilst suffering from suicidal mania. The jury wasted little time in finding him 'not guilty on the ground of insanity'.[43] His admission notes at Holloway attributed his insanity to 'intemperance and residence in a hot climate'; he had travelled widely during his long and relatively successful career as a navel engineer. [44]

There were also occasions when new patients at Holloway prompted the superintendent to voice concerns about their poor mental and physical condition, describing them as 'feeble' and 'moribund'.[45] Rees Philipps repeatedly stated that both the age of some newly admitted patients and the length of time that they had had been either inadequately or totally untreated greatly hindered their potential for recovery or even totally eliminated any such possibility.[46] This suggests that some families may have delayed residential treatment, perhaps seeing institutionalized care as the very last resort for personal and financial reasons. There was also the associated stigma. But, however well intentioned, (or not), such delays adversely affected the patient's mental and physical health. At the onset of mental impairment, families often tried to care for their relatives at home with or without additional assistance. Another option was to board them out nearby with a private nurse, or send them to small private licensed houses where, arguably, the available medical treatment ultimately proved inadequate and failed to produce a cure. Patients who arrived at Holloway 'sparsely nourished' were quickly fed additional supplements to build them up, including beef teas and milk and brandy; any subsequent weight gain was proudly recorded in the patients' notes and was seen as indicative of their being on the road to recovery (see the chapter on therapeutics, pp. 41–65).

At Holloway, patients' families and friends were more likely to have been both actively involved and influential over the committal and discharge of their relatives than at Brookwood. This resulted partially from a class-based confidence, and also that many contributed financially; customers generally demand assurance of an effective service. This makes the abundance of Brookwood families' letters even more surprising. Unlike at Brookwood, a rates-supported institution, Holloway's management operated an active policy of encouraging patient's families to stay at the sanatorium for short periods whilst their relatives underwent treatment. Special accommodation was offered within the beautifully maintained grounds, so that the families could satisfy themselves that the best treatment and most appropriate levels of care were being provided. As shown, most Holloway patients were brought directly from their home and there is some evidence in the patient case books that families remained continually involved with the patients' welfare, although insufficient personal correspondence has survived to fully corroborate this.[47] Many letters written by the patients were never despatched; they were subjected to management censorship and were appended to their case notes as evidence of their continued insanity. This practice was less evident in the Brookwood case books, possibly due to the inmates having little free time within a structured asylum regime, as well as lower literacy levels and the scarcity of writing materials.

As with the Brookwood correspondence, the surviving Holloway letters suggest many reasons why they had not been despatched. At both asylums there were a number of letters which appear lucid and logical, so that the reason for censorship is unclear. Others were rambling or clearly contained examples of delusional thought, threats or obscenities. Letters which were critical of the sanatorium may offer some clues as to why they had not been posted. Such criticism may have been viewed as delusional and therefore an indication of continued instability – it certainly was not good publicity. Some patients realized that their letters did not reach the intended destination. Henry Y. E., a 22-year-old clerk from Hampton Hill with a history of exhibiting 'a great sense of sexual perversion', was admitted to Holloway Sanatorium on 25 January 1886 in an allegedly suicidal condition after having acted 'with the greatest violence' towards his father. Once in the sanatorium, he confessed to the superintendent that he did not feel suicidal but that he had made this claim in order to gain attention.[48] One month after his admission, he wrote to a female friend in the USA and poured out his frustration with his current situation:

> The worst has happened. I am in a lunatic asylum but I am perfectly sane only miserable. I will tell you how I came here. About 5 weeks ago I was insulted by my father & I lost my temper & struck him. For this my mother persuaded me to come to St Ann's Heath, which is the name of this lunatic asylum, Oh, the horror of the place. Can you picture me shut up here? Very shady practices go on in this place, and there are a number of people who have nothing the matter with them, except they have peculiar religious ideas, & their friends shut them up to get rid of them. I have been subject to the most awful indignities. I have to sleep in a room with about 9 other fellows. I have to bath before a host of fellows, and if I am not civil I am locked up in close confinement. Oh the anguish I have suffered. My letters are tampered with & held back & I can get no redress. I am sending this secretly so I do hope you will receive it. I implore you my only friend to pray for me in that I may be released from this awful prison.

This young man's continual disagreements with his father which culminated in the incident described, together with the son's associated guilt, had enabled his mother to persuade him to undergo medical examinations which had ultimately led to his certification and admission to Holloway. In such a way, the sanatorium's management demonstrated their capacity to offer a temporary solution to family disputes and – arguably – provide respite for all involved. Levels of corroboration between the medical profession and the patients' families was often evident; relatives and friends saw the potential for the asylum to become what Coleborne identified as a refuge; an arbiter or practical response to persistent familial difficulties.[49]

This particular young man was perfectly aware that his earlier correspondence had been scrutinized by the authorities. His letter continued:

> I have written imploringly to my mother to ask her to let me free but they won't. I have already written twice before to you from this infernal prison – Did you receive them? If so you will be surprised at their contents. The fact is some of my letters are opened & I could not write what I wanted to. I am sending this note in secret by the kindness of one of the Housemaids.

This housemaid may have been loyal to her employers or she was simply caught out but the letter was intervened and appended to his case notes as evidence of his lunacy. He had no previous medical history nor were there any bad behaviour or overt indications of insanity recorded during his stay, other than his criticism of the sanatorium and referral to 'shady practices'. He was discharged as recovered on 26 March, just two months after his admission.[50]

Usually the family circumstances surrounding patient admissions are unclear, but some indicate underlying problems and tensions of some severity. One father brought both his daughters, aged nineteen and twenty-one years, to the sanatorium just within a few months of each other. The elder, Winifred H. D., was first admitted as a boarder in 1898 for a three-month period, and was then readmitted as a certified patient one month later. She remained at Holloway for a further fourteen months.[51] Her younger sister, Elizabeth, spent just over a year in Holloway. Prior to arriving at the sanatorium in November 1899, she had been cared for in a cottage by a private nurse. Her admission notes states that her father had petitioned for her certification due to a number of unacceptable behaviour patterns that included 'foolish gestures when walking', in addition to extreme restlessness, stripping off her clothing in public places, incoherent conversation, and her 'confessed inability to understand her relationship with her father'. Elizabeth's mother corroborated her husband's evidence and added that their daughter had always been excitable and neurotic.[52]

As seen at the Sussex private asylum at Ticehurst, both male and female patients were referred to Holloway by (usually) male members of their family. Unsurprisingly, reflecting the social and legal norm of nineteenth-century England, most married women were referred by their husbands, although fathers, brothers and male cousins and brothers-in-law were also named petitioners for their female relatives, whether they were married or single.[53]

The evidence provided by family members to the doctors was crucial in order to obtain an accurate assessment of the patient's insanity, and suggests a level of mutual co-operation. There were many reasons why families took steps to have their relatives confined, not least, as Charlotte MacKenzie has pointed out, that the removal of a difficult family member could restore family harmony, albeit temporarily.[54] It is overly simplistic to suggest that husbands and other relatives routinely used asylums to dispose of unwanted individuals such as the elderly or unmarried females. As seen (above), it must be remembered that there is a great deal of evidence from patients' letters and casebook notes which showed that many families, of all classes, cared deeply about their unwell relatives, sought custodial care as a last resort and wanted only reassurance and guidance from the asylum doctors and staff.

There is no evidence of patients coming to Holloway directly from any workhouses, but the records of one woman, Susan B., showed that she had previously spent time in an unspecified workhouse, prior to being brought from home to the sanatorium in 1887 by a female relative or friend. Her first certification occurred in 1883, but it is unclear if her time in the workhouse had been due to her insanity or had resulted from her penury prior to her uncle (Major B.) and the female friend taking over the responsibility for her care.[55] Only a very small number of patients was occasionally transferred from (and to) county asylums, such as Hanwell, Northampton and Glamorgan County asylums. However, most patients came either from other private institutions such as Camberwell House, Peckham House or smaller places such as Brandenburg House, Hammersmith or the nearby Halliford House in Sunbury-on-Thames. Some had previously resided at the charitable St Andrew's Hospital (Northampton).[56] Very occasionally Holloway patients were transferred to Brookwood Asylum, usually due to non-payment of fees. Ellen B. arrived at the sanatorium in June 1899, accompanied by her father from the family home in Kew, Surrey. She had previously made several attempts at suicide and upon arrival she was diagnosed as suffering from 'adolescent melancholia'. She gradually improved during her stay so that the suicidal caution was removed, but following a family visit in January 1900, she relapsed, becoming overly emotional and incoherent which was 'probably due to some very injudicious remarks made to her by her brother on his visit a few days ago'.[57] On 30 March, she was transferred to Brookwood, 'her friends not being able to continue their payments'.[58]

Holloway regularly took in a small number of individuals from the After-Care Association, partially as a result of the hospital's charitable status, but also because Rees Philipps was a trustee on the charity's board. It could be argued that the sanatorium's charitable image was enhanced amongst philanthropic and medical circles by this connection, not to mention amongst the general public, prospective patients and their families[59] Restoring discharged patients to suitable employment was one of the association's key aims.[60] These patients found temporary employment and support not only at the sanatorium, but also in private convalescent homes and other asylums across the country, and even in Romania.[61] Between twenty and twenty-five discharged asylum patients came to stay at Holloway each year via the After-Care Association and were given medical attention, accommodation, food, clothing and money. Although not strictly classed as admissions, these After-Care Association cases participated in sanatorium life; they came from all walks of life and were not all of middle-class origin. Those who were, however, were allowed to associate more freely with the Holloway patients, while the rest were boarded with the staff. There were mixed benefits for the sanatorium; some individuals were useful and made an active contribution to daily life, while others were a source of expense. This group of patients, to some extent, demonstrates the fluidity of 'class' as defined within Holloway's admissions policy.

The Patients' Physical and Mental Condition

Many physically weak and undernourished patients who arrived at Brookwood were potentially long-term chronic patients with little or no prospect of cure. Some of the more extreme cases died within weeks, or even hours, of admission and although these patients had primarily originated from workhouses, this was not always the case. Often patients were filthy and disease-ridden, all indicative of the severe social distress that accompanied unemployment and poverty. Their condition could not be solely accounted for by the possibility of families being inept or uncaring. Very weak patients received special dietary supplements to build them up and both restoratives and purgatives were administered in turn. Holloway's attendants did not usually have to cope with patients ravaged by poverty, but, occasionally, they dealt with medical conditions that required special attention. Some Holloway patients had also been severely neglected by relatives and there were reports of a few patients arriving at Holloway in an unkempt condition, or with bruising, and on one or two occasions, with fractures. General paralysis of the insane (GPI) dogged the populations of both asylums and, depending on the progress of the disease, undermined the patients' physical health, including their mobility and physical strength. Seen as a complication of insanity, GPI was characterized by a combination of symptoms such as progressive dementia, often accompanied by grandiose delusions, failing memory, facial tremors, slurred speech and uncertain gait.[62] Patients allegedly suffering from GPI were frequently 'dirty' (incontinent) and this, combined with the symptoms given above, impaired patient independence so that constant medical attention was required.[63]

Many medical practitioners identified the connection between mental illness and physical deprivation and saw this as a 'moral cause' of insanity.[64] The relationship between deprivation and insanity was acknowledged by Brushfield, when, in 1888, he remarked upon the current economic downturn in trade and agriculture that had, in his opinion, greatly influenced 'the character of insanity'. This meant fewer acute and relatively curable cases, but a corresponding increase in the number of the 'melancholic and demented' being admitted to the asylum.[65] A large proportion of patients originated from the poorest parts of South London and was subject to inadequate housing and irregular (and physically harsh) employment, although equally, poverty was no stranger to the countryside. In this study, both physical and mental illnesses connected with poverty were more likely to be associated with Brookwood than Holloway patients. The proportion varied, but, for example, in 1868, nearly half of all the admissions to Brookwood were described as being physically 'weak or bad'.[66] The same issues were still seen as worthy of comment sixteen years later but on this occasion, the superintendent was relieved to be able to report that despite 'the large number of feeble & broken down cases imported into the asylum', the general health of the inmates had remained good and there had been no outbreak of any contagious diseases.[67] Some care should be exercised in assuming that in the later years, admissions of feeble and ill patients continued at the same levels; in 1881, for example, the records show that the majority of men and women (just over 70 per cent) were described as in fair, moderate or even good health. How these terms were defined by the medical staff at that time is difficult to ascertain, however; 'Fair' was the description applied to one patient with phthisis, and 'Good' to another who suffered from heart disease.[68]

When a patient arrived at Brookwood, as part of the diagnostic process an attempt was made to identify a supposed cause for insanity which was recorded in the registers, along with the patients' personal details.[69] The cause, however, remained elusive in many cases. 'Business worries' or 'anxiety about work' were regularly ascribed to (predominantly) male patients, reflecting the connection between assured income and mental well-being. John M., a 35-year-old carpenter, was admitted to Brookwood in 1871from the London parish of St Saviour's as a result of his mania bought about by 'want of regular employment'. Richard H., 52, lost his position as a restaurant manager in 1891 and was admitted later that year suffering from dementia, allegedly due to his fear of poverty. Whilst largely associated with the male patients, some women were also deeply affected by employment issues and those without male support were especially vulnerable. Sarah C. was a 52-year-old spinster whose melancholia and subsequent three-year stay in Brookwood from 1881 was believed to have been caused by her 'Want of success in her occupation' which was described as 'Letter of lodgings', a popular way for self-supporting women to earn an income at this time. Harriet R., 44, had previously worked as a servant, but her husband's desertion precipitated her mania so that she was incarcerated in August 1871, in a weak and enfeebled physical condition.[70]

Of course, Holloway patients were not immune to pecuniary difficulties and business-related anxieties, although, according to the admissions registers, these appear to be relatively few and were often attended by other 'causes' such as intemperance or religious excitement. Evidence of overt poverty is rare in the surviving Holloway data, although many patients had suffered reduced circumstances and so applied for charitable assistance with their fees. Some cases were allegedly related to general anxiety combined with overwork and excessive studying. Frank H., a 32-year-old stock jobber from Finchley, was brought to the sanatorium by his brother in September 1889, suffering from delusional insanity brought on by business worries. He remained there until his death in 1944. In February 1893, Emily H., a married 'gentlewoman' of fifty-two years of age arrived suffering from melancholia due to unspecified money losses but she was discharged as recovered just over one year later. Both of these patients had been admitted in good bodily health.[71]

Infectious diseases were also associated with poverty and malnutrition; it was not unusual for such conditions as diarrhoea or influenza to spread quickly through the packed asylum where there were many weak and susceptible patients. For example, in 1871 a female metropolitan workhouse patient was cited as the source of a severe outbreak of smallpox in Brookwood.[72] The disease attacked attendants and patients alike but was able to be mainly confined to the female division. Unlike anything that occurred at Holloway, a huge vaccination programme was undertaken that included all the patients, staff and any workmen and tradespeople who visited the asylum on a regular basis.[73] This, and other measures, for example banning relatives from visiting for two months, segregating religious services and using copious amounts of disinfectant, were all speedily implemented to restrict the spread of disease.[74]

Although these are examined more fully in the chapter on therapeutics, it should be noted that the principal mental illnesses (mania, melancholia and dementia), together with their variations, were found at both Brookwood and Holloway. At Brookwood, almost 50 per cent of the patients admitted of both sexes were diagnosed as suffering from mania, whilst melancholia accounted for slightly less than 33 per cent. Dementia was attributed to 15 per cent of males and 21 per cent of females. The available data from the Holloway records shows a similar distribution of these primary diseases.[75] Some patients suffered from anxiety and delusions about food, so that they refused to eat, behaviour which was less common amongst Brookwood patients.[76]

Patients with specific medical requirements perceived as relevant to mental disorders, such as epilepsy or GPI, were also admitted to both asylums. GPI was usually attended by chronic trembling and brain disease and led to eventual death. Other symptoms included unsteady gait, delusions and dirty habits. This particular disease was frequently diagnosed in male asylum patients. Later it was understood to be associated with the advanced stages of syphilitic infection, but it has been suggested that as the diagnosis became more precise towards the end of the nineteenth century, this corresponded with a slight decline in numbers as the use of the term became more restricted.[77]

By the mid-1870s, 25 per cent of all workhouse patients sent to Brookwood were reportedly either epileptic or syphilitic. The nature of their conditions meant that they were difficult cases that required intense care and supervision, and were thus hastily despatched by workhouse masters in order to save resources and maintain order, as acknowledged in the superintendents' reports. These patients were often described as 'dangerous' and/or 'suicidal' but given the relatively low number of 'accidents' that occurred at Brookwood, such labelling must be viewed with a degree of contextual sensitivity. The usage of these terms expedited the removal of unwanted patients from the workhouses and released space for more desirable and easily managed cases.[78] Conversely, Brushfield was vehement in his condemnation of the alleged workhouse practice of detaining the quieter and less troublesome inmates for much longer than necessary before obtaining the required certification for their transferral to the asylum, which minimized or even totally eradicated their chances of recovering. Brushfield declared that this practice occurred even when there were plenty of available beds at Brookwood so that there was no justifiable reason for the workhouse not to apply for their removal.[79]

In keeping with asylum administration at the time, Brushfield dealt with many competing priorities, but keeping the patients safe was at the heart of asylum management. Suicidal, homicidal and epileptic patients all required additional supervision but there was one small but significant group of patients that was of particular concern: the children.

Children and Adolescent Admissions

The admission of a small number of children and adolescent patients to both Brookwood Asylum and Holloway Sanatorium was problematic to the respective managements, as these young patients required specialized and appropriate care that the asylums struggled to make available. Young children were mostly brought to Brookwood by their parents, who were often distraught and exhausted with caring for children who had not developed as expected. Although no such young children were admitted to Holloway, adolescents were admitted to both institutions with a wide range of seemingly difficult behaviours, including overt sexual awareness and challenging adult authority. Rees Phillips had direct experience of working with children during his earlier career, though he had not yet been required to put this to great use while at the sanatorium.[80]

Occasionally babies were born to female patients at Brookwood and these were quickly separated from their mothers; two pregnant women admitted in 1869 subsequently gave birth and one baby was sent to the workhouse, and the other returned to the husband.[81] As pointed out by Melling, Adair and Forsythe, recent scholarship regarding the role of the family in the committal process has omitted to explore the admission of children to asylums following the 1845 legislation.[82] Earlier research by Parry-Jones showed that between 1815 and 1895, Bethlem alone had admitted over a thousand children and adolescents. The county asylum at Exminster admitted an average of 1.5 children per year, a low figure attributed to the rising numbers of adult admissions.[83] Worcester County Asylum admitted 195 children between 1854 and 1900.[84] Estimates of the actual numbers of children being admitted to asylums across England and Wales vary, but suggest that an average of two or three children under fourteen years of age were admitted each year, which increased slightly as the nineteenth century drew to a close.[85]

At Brookwood, six children between the ages of nine and fifteen were resident by 1869.[86] Unlike at Exminster, the data collected for Brookwood shows
slightly more children admitted during the selected years, six girls and five boys
in total. Four children were admitted in 1871, only one in 1881, but six in 1891,
indicating that the considerable rise in adult admissions did not preclude the
admission of often very small children.[87] Henry E. was only four years of age
when he arrived at Brookwood in December 1891. Described as an 'idiot' from
the first year of his life, he only stayed two months before he was transferred to
another institution. Many children were described in case books as being congenital idiots or imbeciles and often they suffered additional physical handicaps,
like eleven-year-old Anne T., who was blind from birth.[88]

Children were usually brought in by their parents although they were
sometimes transferred from the workhouse infirmary, or more rarely, other institutions. Such was the case of Mary Jane S. who in November 1875, at the age of
five, was transferred to Brookwood, having already spent thirteen months of her
short life in Fisherton House, Salisbury. Described in her Brookwood case notes
as a 'congenital idiot', her medical certificate gave the reasons for her incarceration from such a young age:

> She is very mischievous and destructive and might be dangerous to other children
> in the same Ward, as she is very active and strong for her age. She is very deficient in
> intellectual capacity, but can articulate a few words such as 'Mamma, Dada' and will if
> urged attempt others, she is entirely restless, never still when dressed and about, for a
> moment, running fearlessly or blindly against any obstacles and frequently bruising &
> knocking herself, of which she has several superficial marks on her person & requiring
> the upmost watchfulness to prevent her receiving serious injury.[89]

In 1877, her mother wrote to the superintendent asking to visit her daughter;
this was at a time when the asylum was effectively closed to the outside world
whilst trying to eradicate an outbreak of smallpox:

> Sir
>   Please oblige by sending word if my little girl Mary Jane S. is in good health and
> if there is any difference in her mental state. Please say if she may be visited. I do not
> hear of any cases of Smallpox or know of any. Her father would like to see her and
> would feel obliged by an answer before Tuesday.
>   I think my little girl might learn the Dumb Alphabet reading and writing but I
> suppose in that case she would require to be removed from Brookwood to an asylum
> for children thus marked & must leave to your discretion.[90]

It is not possible to confirm if the visit took place or indeed, how many times her
parents saw her before she was eventually transferred to Darenth Asylum on 6
August 1880. Only three days earlier, she had been assaulted by a patient in the
ward.[91] There is no evidence to suggest that the youngest Brookwood patients

were allowed any visiting concessions on account of their age; as with childhood physical illnesses, there was no stated belief in the value of parent-and-child contact even in the best family circumstances.[92]

As might be expected, many of the children admitted to general asylums suffered from mental retardation ('idiots'), but some were epileptic, psychotic or just exhibited behavioural difficulties that their families were perhaps unable, or unwilling, to manage. The diagnosis of moral insanity was equally likely to be applied to children as to adults; this was later adapted to 'moral imbecility', and in this guise was responsible over many years for the compulsory admission of children with a wide range of problems that ranged from retardation, or conduct disorders, to promiscuity or autism.[93]

In the emergent psychiatric profession, the notion of segregation from familiar surroundings was seen to be just as important for children as it was for adults. Once separated from family and friends and placed among strangers, the belief was that the child would 'be obliged to conform to the rules of the house and carry out the treatment which has been ordered'.[94] In 1867, the 'imbecile' Elizabeth K., with her almost unintelligible speech, was first admitted to Brookwood at the age of nine. Already the subject of institutional care, she had been transferred from Bethnal House where she had been for a few months. During her three-year stay at Brookwood, she was reported to have quietened down, and had learnt the rudiments of cards and other games in between being put to work scrubbing the wards. Unfortunately, Elizabeth was attacked on several occasions by adult patients. In May 1870 she was discharged as recovered, but readmitted a year later as her violent behaviour had returned, as testified by her mother; a not-untypical example of active parent co-operation in sending their children to the asylum. Her Brookwood case notes indicate that there was some limited success in managing her bouts of violence by such methods as isolating her in a padded cell, using shower baths and administering some chemical therapy. However, her difficult behaviour was never completely eradicated and two years later she was transferred to Hanwell Asylum.[95]

Annie S. was only ten when she was transferred to Brookwood from Richmond Workhouse; in her certificate, her congenital insanity was attributed to a fall, although the asylum case notes also acknowledged that it was more likely to have been the result of a defect from birth. There was also the possibility that hereditary influences may have played a part as her father had reportedly committed suicide. She resided at Brookwood from 1890 to 1893 when she died from an epileptic fit.[96] Epilepsy was a condition that, understandably, many parents struggled to manage; the parents of four-year-old Maxwell E. described his constant and dangerous mobility, exacerbated by his frequent epileptic fits, that led them to seek institutional care. He was brought to Brookwood in 1891 but –

regretting their decision – his father successfully petitioned for the return of his son to the family only a few months later.[97]

Death was the most likely outcome for these children. Five-year-old Albert H., a congenital and epileptic imbecile, was transferred from Kingston Workhouse in January 1891 but only survived at Brookwood for just under a year; the cause of death was given as exhaustion from fits.[98] Other children spent several years at Brookwood; eleven-year-old Frederick B., who suffered from imbecility and epilepsy, arrived in June 1867, having spent the previous four years at Wandsworth at the request of his mother. He remained at Brookwood until his death in 1875.[99]

Public asylums were fully aware of the difficulties associated with accommodating children; the very young ones were initially kept in the female block at Brookwood where the patients often (but not always) took them under their wing. Adolescents (over twelve years of age) were placed in the appropriate adult wards. This practice echoed that which was carried out in general hospitals prior to the advent of special wards, and later, hospitals, for children.[100] In 1884, Brookwood's superintendent aired the problem of appropriate accommodation and its impact on the children's potential:

> Among those sent to the Union were two girls, aged respectively ten and twelve years, who had been admitted during the year. Both of these were congenitally deficient, and were stated to be very troublesome and dangerous to others, but proved, with a little management, to be quiet, tractable, and docile, and to possess a certain amount of intelligence. The associations of an ordinary lunatic ward are very bad for such children, as they pick up objectionable habits with greater facility, and it is to be regretted that they cannot be either retained in the Workhouse or sent to an Institution where they could be properly trained.[101]

Acknowledging the lack of any option other than placing the children with the adult female lunatics, Brookwood's management and the Commissioners in Lunacy both articulated the urgent need for specialized accommodation for these young patients. Those that had been transferred from the workhouses were often particularly difficult to control and were potentially a danger to themselves or to others. Families were driven to despair in their attempts to care for them, often struggling in very difficult social circumstances with other children to consider and protect.

In 1895, there were seventeen children (under the age of sixteen) in custody at Brookwood, all of whom were described as being 'idiots and imbeciles' and whom the superintendent believed would be better cared for in a separate establishment.[102] By this time, the few idiot children remaining at Brookwood had at least been segregated from the adult patients in dedicated small rooms located in both the female and male wing where they were reportedly 'well off for toys'.[103]

Alternatives for children and young people suffering from idiocy other than the county asylum gradually emerged, so that it became increasingly possible to remove them from the ordinary wards to specialized care, although accommodating the numbers was an ongoing problem.[104] The charitable Earlswood Asylum, which also admitted a percentage of private patients, had opened in 1847, and later, the superintendent, Dr Langdon Down, opened his private Normansfield Hospital in 1868, a larger institution that was able to care for 140 patients by 1898.[105] With annual fees of £100 to £200, it was the wealthier families who were able to send their children to such an establishment.

By way of contrast, unlike Brookwood, there were very few child or adolescent admissions to Holloway. The youngest patients were fifteen years of age when admitted; one young German girl in 1893 and later, another girl, Ella C., arrived at the sanatorium in 1899. Her certificate stated that her insanity was caused by sunstroke at the age of four. She was brought to the sanatorium from the family home in Wiltshire accompanied by her father. She was in a severely undernourished state; whether this had resulted from neglect or not is unknown, but upon admission she was diagnosed as suffering from rickets. She was fifteen years of age but due to her physical condition, she was described as resembling a girl of eight or nine years old. Whilst in the sanatorium, she remained in a stupor for several months and had to be tube-fed by the nurses. By the time she was discharged back to her family four months later, she was able to talk more coherently and had gained a substantial 30 lb in weight.[106]

These children were a small, but important and consistent, percentage of the many patients admitted to these two asylums each year, especially at Brookwood. Despite the lack of appropriate accommodation, it seems that, at least initially, the management was either relatively happy to admit these children, or did not discourage the practice, while recognizing the need for specialized accommodation. This was partially due to the growing awareness and acceptance of ideas of hereditary insanity amongst the psychiatric profession, and the belief in the necessity of the earliest possible intervention. For example, in 1873, Henry Maudsley stated: 'the insane individual represents the beginning of a degeneracy which if not checked will go on from generation to generation and end finally in the extreme degeneracy of idiocy'.[107] The seemingly under-recorded presence of children – mostly 'imbeciles' or 'idiots' from birth – in nineteenth-century county asylums offers future opportunities to examine the care that was provided for these children prior to the creation of specialized accommodation.

Conclusion

This chapter has introduced the patients of Brookwood Asylum and Holloway Sanatorium. Their origins, and their previous treatment – or lack thereof – affected their physical and mental condition and had important implications for their eventual cure. The outcome helped to define what contemporaries understood as their 'success' in caring for and treating their patients.[108]

The families of the middle- and upper-class Holloway patients were more likely to have been directly involved in the admission and discharge process, by virtue of their superior education and 'consumer' status. This empowered them to demand high standards and allowed them, to some extent, to influence the course of patient care. The extensive facilities allowed them to be active in the care of their loved ones.

More surprising is the evidence from the Brookwood records, in particular the personal letters, which demonstrates that the families of the less well-off and pauper patients did not merely succumb to medical hegemony to the extent that they 'gave up' their relatives to the specialists. The surviving letters bear testimony to the varied and very real concerns of friends and family and their desire for news and information. They collaborated with the doctors, but this did not necessarily mean that they absolved themselves of all responsibility, although they did not always wish to be held accountable for discharged relatives whose return could affect their standard of living.[109]

At Brookwood, surprisingly consistent numbers of young children were admitted, whereas, at Holloway, only a small number of adolescents were traced. It is clear that Brookwood's management was very uncomfortable with the initial arrangements, which meant admitting vulnerable youngsters into the potentially threatening environment of the adult wards. The management repeatedly advocated separate institutions for mentally disordered children.[110]

Brookwood, and other large county institutions, were primarily intended to serve the insane poor, but the reality was more nuanced. Similarly, the patient population at Holloway Sanatorium did not conform to the original intentions of its founder. The composition of the populations of both asylums will be examined in-depth in the next chapter, allowing an analysis of trends and themes within the admission and discharge procedures that, to some extent, challenge the previous historiography regarding alleged Victorian class and gender discrimination.

4 'HURRY, WORRY, ANNOYANCE AND NEEDLESS TROUBLE': PATIENTS IN RESIDENCE

Introduction

This chapter uses the surviving admissions and discharge data of both institutions to analyse the characteristics of the patients and explore the treatment outcomes: why men and women found themselves incarcerated, why some never left alive, and the reasons yet others were discharged very soon after admission. These details allow us to consider whether Poor Law institutions such as Brookwood Asylum were representative 'microcosms of society', or whether they held only its poorest and most disruptive members.[1] Challenging the stereotypical reputation of the nineteenth-century asylum, there is no evidence here to show that more women were deliberately detained than men. Both Brookwood and Holloway Sanatorium admitted approximately equal numbers of the sexes, which supports those historians who contradict Showalter's *The Female Malady*.[2] Male and female patients *were* diagnosed with different illnesses, and the research here indicates that women *did* tend to stay longer in the asylum than their male counterparts, but the latter could be a matter of choice, especially for middle-class women.

Holloway's management would have presumed that the vast majority of applicants were intrinsically 'middle-class', taking into account not only their financial circumstances but also broader social indicators of status. Lorraine Walsh has suggested that, when considering the asylum patient's experience, there is the potential to overlook the importance of other factors beyond class concerns, such as contemporary interpretations of respectability and socially acceptable behaviour, which were the cornerstones of moral therapy.[3] Further, it is not enough to suggest that private asylums simply favoured wealthy patients while the poor were restricted to the public system.[4] While Walsh has used the example of the Dundee Royal (a mixed institution), the research on Brookwood and Holloway goes some way to endorsing this view, despite their obvious financial and managerial differences. As seen in Devon, the diagnosis and subsequent detention of the insane rested on an evaluation of their social and personal status together with their resources, subsequently validated by medical and legal mechanisms.[5]

Patient Admissions to Brookwood

During the first thirty years, a total of 8,891 patients were admitted to Brookwood for treatment. From 1867 to 1891 admissions continued to rise each year and peaked in 1876 when 451 patients were admitted, and again in 1884 with 585 new cases (Figure 4.1).[6] By 1870, the asylum had reached capacity so that until 1874 inclusive, general admissions were comparatively low (less than two hundred per year). Remedial building work was undertaken and while in progress, this severely disrupted the asylum's daily routine as well as restricting the intake of new patients. By 1890, the completion of a variety of building projects, together with the county's administrative and boundary changes meant that Brookwood admitted 394 patients that year, although this decreased the following year and levelled out until the end of the century. By 1900, Brookwood was a large institution with a daily average of 1,033 resident patients.

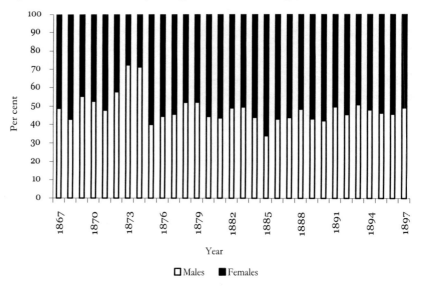

Figure 4.1: Brookwood Asylum, general patient admissions by sex, 1867–97. Source: Brookwood Patient Admissions Registers, Surrey History Centre.

This large number of admissions strained Brookwood's resources. The medical superintendent reported an ongoing demand for accommodation and that his wards were filled to capacity. Nevertheless, considering the volume of patients, the asylum maintained a relatively good safety record, with infrequent accidents and suicides. This represented a considerable achievement for the asylum's management. Relapsed cases, or readmissions to Brookwood, stood at roughly 5 per cent over the years, which Brushfield stated to be 'about one half of the general average in English County Asylums'.[7] This he attributed to the asylum's thorough and careful discharge strategy. Usually, patients were initially released on a month's trial, personal circumstances were investigated, and their families were issued with a leaflet that contained practical guidance to help avoid relapse. This included advice on diet and rest, advocated the restriction of stimulants such as beer and opium, and cautioned that 'hurry, worry, annoyance, and needless trouble' could hinder a complete and lasting recovery.[8]

Admissions to Brookwood Asylum during the first thirty years after opening (1867–97) show little significant difference between the numbers of male and female patients: women were not over-represented amongst the admissions and they broadly reflected the county's demographic profile. On average, men accounted for 47 per cent of the total number of patients admitted, and women accounted for 53 per cent, a ratio that was similar to other asylums at the time. At the Buckinghamshire County Asylum, as at Brookwood, 53 per cent of the admissions were female, reflecting the population ratios of both counties.[9] The Devon Asylum mirrors this proportion, and at Leicestershire County Asylum 54 per cent of the paupers admitted between 1860 and 1865 were female.[10] This situation was not unique to England; in his work on South Carolina Asylum, Peter McCandless demonstrated that, before 1900, there was very little difference between the admission figures for male and female patients and in some years, men outnumbered women.[11] Of course, some individual years varied; women accounted for as little as 27 per cent of Brookwood admissions in 1873, as high as 60 per cent in 1875 and 1884, often dependent on the availability of beds. In years that there was more accommodation for both sexes, general admissions also increased.[12] Even when female admissions did increase slightly, this to some extent reflects the county's male-to-female ratio; the 1871 census showed that, for every 1,000 men in Surrey, there were 1,115 women.[13]

Neither men nor women were more likely to be readmitted to Brookwood. Relapsed cases of both sexes were usually patients who had been released following persistent requests from friends and relatives. They were sometimes discharged against the better judgement of the medical staff, who suspected that, occasionally, relatives' motives were less than honourable. The patient may have been of some practical use to the family or they wanted their release because of 'some more mercenary motive'.[14] Nearly all readmitted cases were reported to have returned to Brookwood in a worse condition than when they left. On average, relapsed patients remained outside the asylum for less than a year.[15]

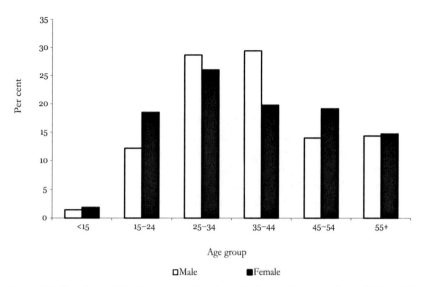

Figure 4.2: **Brookwood Asylum, general patient admissions by age and sex, 1871, 1881 and 1891. Source: Brookwood Patient Admissions Registers, Surrey History Centre.**

The data for Brookwood represented in Figure 4.2 is taken from a sample of the three census years (1871, 1881 and 1891), and shows that more women than men were admitted from the younger and older age groups.[16] With regards to male admissions, a greater proportion were in the 25–44 age group, comprising a significant number of 'difficult' young men who were transferred from south London workhouses. At both asylums, the proportion of females to males in the over 45s age group was greater, indicating that, to some extent regardless of social class, there were limited options for women believed to be suffering from mental illness particularly as they were seen as unmarriageable and unlikely to bear children.

Despite legislative assumptions regarding their earning power, poor women were often major contributors to the family income by direct and indirect means.[17] The working-class woman would arguably have had less time to consider her emotional or psychological problems, although this is not a scientifically valid reason for fewer of them in these age groups being admitted to Brookwood. Many women were solely responsible for young families, partially due to their longer life expectancy, yet others had been deserted by their husbands, or economic necessity had obliged the menfolk to leave home to seek temporary or seasonal work elsewhere.[18] Provided their condition was not too severe, mentally or physically defective women of virtually any age were often maintained at home where they were able to perform useful domestic tasks and take care of children whilst other family members were out at work.

Young single men, aged 16–35, comprised the vast majority of male work-house patients admitted to Brookwood; some years they accounted for up to three-quarters of all male admissions. On average, only 6 per cent of male admissions from the workhouse were recorded as being married. These younger men were usually alleged to be maniacal and difficult to control, and if their certificates described them as being dangerous and/or suicidal, they were unable to remain in the workhouse for longer than two weeks. Cost was a strong consideration; however, transfers also reflected the ability of any one particular workhouse to control its lunatics.[19] Discipline was always a workhouse priority and larger unions (such as Lambeth) built special wards to cater for potentially difficult young men and women in an attempt to minimize general disruption.[20] Despite the establishment of county asylums, workhouses remained important providers of accommodation for the insane; up to 25 per cent of pauper lunatics resided in workhouses, a figure that increased from 3,829 (1844) to 17,825 (1890).[21]

Both Brookwood and Holloway cared for a wide range of patients suffering illnesses that varied in their severity – from neurosis to those with serious mental disorders. As Hilary Marland has highlighted, doctors recognized that poor women were not exempt from experiencing difficult and upsetting emotions associated with their roles as housewives and mothers, and that worry and hardship could exacerbate these difficulties.[22] In some cases, hereditary factors were believed to cause or make a patient more vulnerable to mental illness, particularly when there were other pressures. Louisa P. had experienced several previous attacks believed to have been hereditary in origin. She had been treated at other institutions, but the attack which occurred in April 1881 was attributed to her confinement two weeks before her admission to Brookwood. At home, her symptoms of insanity had appeared within a few days of the birth. Sadly, her baby died, which quickly escalated her condition so that the family took urgent action:

> she became very maniacal, violent and spiteful, and her husband was obliged to remove her to the union in the middle of the night where she has been very noisy and troublesome and at times violent and suicidal and last night tried to strangle herself.[23]

Patient Admissions to Holloway

General admissions to the Holloway Sanatorium over a twenty-year period (1885–1905) show that, similar to Brookwood, there was very little difference between the numbers of men and women admitted. Again, the occasional decreases in the female-to-male ratio reflect the lack of available beds whilst building work was in progress so as to meet demand. During the first six months, seventy-three patients and sixteen voluntary boarders were admitted, with seventy remaining at the end of the year. Compared to Brookwood, it remained relatively small; when full towards the end of the century, there was just over one-third of the number incarcerated at the county asylum. But despite being a smaller institution, the private regime was not without its problems, some of which were unique and were directly associated with caring for patients that were generally from higher socio-economic groups.[24]

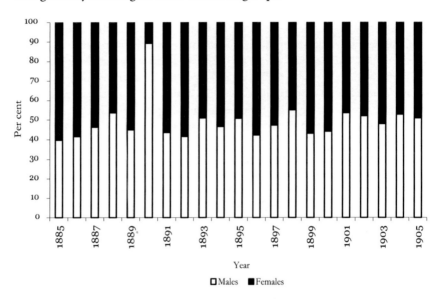

Figure 4.3: Holloway Sanatorium, general patient admissions by sex, 1885–1905, certified patients only. Source: Holloway Admission Registers and Annual Reports, Surrey History Centre.

During the course of the following year (1886), 89 certified patients were admitted and 17 boarders were registered; 110 patients and 9 boarders remained in the asylum on 31 December. Some of the quieter patients were placed in cottages within the sanatorium's grounds where they were cared for by married attendants or, in some instances, other non-medical employees. This practice also occurred at Brookwood, but at Holloway it was arguably more useful, given the smaller scale of the asylum, the high staff-to-patient ratio and the restricted accommodation within the main building.

During the first eighteen months, women accounted for 60 per cent of the total number of patient admissions to Holloway, although this initial surge subsided so that during the first twenty years, female admissions averaged 52 per cent of all admissions, similar to Brookwood. Fluctuations are accounted for by the availability, or not, of accommodation for women; up to 30 per cent more women were admitted in 1892, for example, once more beds had become available.[25] These percentages are also in keeping with those found at other private institutions such as Wonford House.[26] At Holloway, Rees Philipps stated that women were far more prone to insanity than men. However, he alleged that they also demonstrated signs of greater 'recoverability' as their 'nervous organisation is less stable than that of the male and is therefore more liable to merely functional disturbance'.[27] Men were seen to be more likely to suffer from more serious mental ailments and were prone to general paralysis and death. Women's proclivity for recovery, however, did not guarantee their release, as many remained in the sanatorium for long periods of time if they were not discharged within a year of admission.

Due to the limited extant records, it has only been possible to consider data consistently for 1885–90; these do, however, show a different pattern in male and female admissions from that at Brookwood. More men than women under the age of thirty-four were admitted into the sanatorium, but women consistently dominated the admissions for all the age groups over thirty-five years.

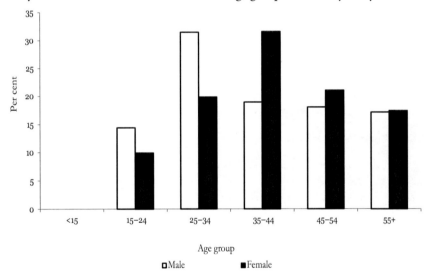

Figure 4.4: Holloway Sanatorium, patient admissions by age and sex, 1885–90, all patients. Source: Holloway Admissions Registers, Surrey History Centre.

The majority of admissions were of patients in the 'middle age groups', i.e. the 25–44 age group. Some years however, older (male and female) patients accounted for a higher percentage of the new intake; for example, in 1890, 52 per cent were aged between forty and ninety years. Rees Philipps believed that this compromised the sanatorium's recovery rate, as it was his opinion that the optimum age for admissions to achieve recovery was twenty to thirty years. Despite the superintendent's seemingly pessimistic view, the sanatorium's recovery rate for 1890 was 55 per cent, the highest rate since opening.[28]

Status and Occupation

Unmarried and widowed patients accounted for most male and female admissions to both Brookwood and Holloway. The data for these three census years (see Table 4.1) clearly shows that the same numbers of male and female patients were admitted to Brookwood. There were equal numbers of married and single women, excluding widows, but there were slightly more single women than single men. Female longevity is again demonstrated by the much higher numbers of widows than widowers. Considerably more married than single men were admitted to Brookwood, suggesting that there were economic imperatives to finding a cure for the family breadwinner.

Table 4.1: Admissions to Brookwood, 1871, 1881 and 1891,
by sex and marital status (per cent).

	Female	Male
N	338	338
Single	42	39
Married	42	55
Widowed	14	4
Unknown/not given	1	2

Source: Brookwood Admissions Registers Surrey History Centre.

In the experience of Brookwood's superintendent, many relatives did not want to care for their harmless lunatics. He pointed to the availability of Caterham Asylum (operational from 1870) which opened in response to the demand for accommodation for the chronic insane and the fact that 'the residents of towns and populous places appear to be adverse to what may be termed the home treatment of their insane relations who are quiet and inoffensive'.[29] This was more likely to be the case with elderly or widowed patients and the higher number of widows admitted suggests a degree of vulnerability, whatever their age, particularly if there were additional physical disabilities. Sarah R., a fur clipper from Bermondsey, was twenty-nine years old when she arrived at Brookwood, having spent the previous six months in St Olave's workhouse. It is unclear how long she had been widowed or if her excessive alcohol consumption had begun prior to or following the loss of her husband. She was deemed a suicide risk, had difficulties with both her speech and with walking and her memory was allegedly defective. These traits, her drinking, and possibly her economic frailty were sufficient reasons for her father-in-law to have brought her case to the attention of the authorities.[30]

Brookwood patient admissions in 1871, 1881 and 1891 show that many men, and some women, had a given occupation and therefore possessed the means to earn a living, although personal circumstances and living standards would have varied. Industrialization had changed class relationships and created a new urbanized and articulate middle class. For both female and male patients, as is common practice, the category of 'unclassified' (as demonstrated in Table 4.2 and Table 4.3) includes all those patients who were referred to in the Brookwood records as 'housewives' or having 'no occupation.'[31]

Direct comparison of the two sexes is difficult as many women (particularly those transferred from the workhouses) did not have an occupation listed in their notes (for example, thirty-one out of eighty-nine admissions in 1891). Nevertheless, it is clear that, on the whole, more male admissions tended to be drawn from the middle classes; overall, 39 per cent of male patients were professionals, managers and skilled workers. The comparable figure for females is nearly half that of the males, 16 per cent. The relatively high percentage of female lower skilled workers can be explained by patients who were previously employed in some form of service (such as domestic servants and laundresses).[32]

Table 4.2: Brookwood female occupations, 1871, 1881 and 1891.

	1871	1881	1891	Total
N	94	137	89	320
Higher managers and professionals	1	2	1	2
Lower managers and professionals, clerical and sales	5	4	6	5
Foremen and skilled workers	15	8	3	9
Farmers and fishermen	0	1	0	0
Lower skilled workers	36	32	30	33
Unskilled workers	19	15	11	15
Lower and unskilled farm and garden workers	5	0	4	3
Unclassified*	18	39	44	34
Total	100	100	100	100

* includes housewives, no occupation, occupation not stated
Source: Brookwood Admissions Registers, Surrey History Centre.

Table 4.3: Brookwood male occupations, 1871, 1881 and 1891.

	1871	1881	1891	Total
N	86	107	88	281
Higher managers and professionals	0	6	3	3
Lower managers and professionals, clerical and sales	17	16	13	15
Foremen and skilled workers	31	19	14	21
Farmers and fishermen	0	0	0	0
Lower skilled workers	13	21	17	17

	1871	1881	1891	Total
Unskilled workers	27	30	24	27
Lower and unskilled farm and garden workers	8	5	18	10
Unclassified*	3	5	11	6
Total	**100**	**100**	**100**	**100**

*   includes no occupation, occupation not stated

Source: Brookwood Admissions Registers, Surrey History Centre.

Arguably, a working-class male was more likely to affect family resources if he was ill and unemployed, and, if he were married and a claimant of poor relief, he was also more visible to the authorities. Families may have been more willing to submit male relatives to medical scrutiny in the hope of obtaining a cure for the breadwinner. Charlotte MacKenzie has explored this in her work on male patients at Ticehurst, where families were prepared to spend considerable sums of money in the hope of procuring a recovery.[33] If this were the case for the comparatively wealthy, then the need to restore the breadwinner to mental stability and competence was even more critical for working-class families.

Most of the men who arrived at Brookwood from the workhouse had previously maintained a former trade or skill, excluding those who were listed as labourers. In 1871, only two men out of the eighty-six who were newly admitted were described as having no occupation. In all, over forty-five different occupations were represented, including carpenter, coachman, groom, omnibus conductor, waterside labourer and wire drawer.[34] Perhaps less predictable were the admissions of a pattern designer, a commission agent and government clerk; men more representative of the class intended for admission to Holloway, thus demonstrating the varied patient culture of these asylums. Occasionally, patients were removed from Brookwood and transferred to a private asylum if family circumstances improved or if relatives suddenly chose to pay for their care. This was the case of one male patient on a special order signed by two of the Commissioners in Lunacy and who was removed from Brookwood to the nearby Holloway Sanatorium in December 1890.[35] (As shown earlier, this process was sometimes reversed, and Holloway patients were transferred to Brookwood when relatives would not or could not pay the fees.)

It was probably not entirely accurate that so many women admitted to Brookwood did not have an occupation, as asylum officials may have ignored certain types of activities. Edward Higgs has shown that women's occupations were frequently under-represented in the nineteenth-century census returns, not least because there was often a reluctance to categorize what was viewed as essentially 'women's work' as an occupation.[36] Amongst those who were regarded as having been in employment, a wide range of female occupations were represented at Brookwood, such as stay maker, fur puller, firework maker and prostitute, together with, more typically, housekeeper, dressmaker, laundress, milliner and field worker.[37] Domestic servants (the largest category of women's employment at this time) accounted for just over 20 per cent of all female admissions ascribed an occupation. Female domestic servants were particularly vulnerable, as many 'lived in'; loss of employment for these women could mean homelessness, destitution and the workhouse. Securing a post without a 'good character' was virtually impossible and references could be withheld by an employer for a variety of (not necessarily valid) reasons. Mary O. C., aged twenty-one, was admitted to Brookwood in February 1881 and was diagnosed with mania. She had spent the previous six days in Camberwell Workhouse where she had been excitable and noisy. Her admission notes to Brookwood allege that that she was 'very hysterical and flighty' but also that her extreme thinness and irregular periods were because 'she has been very hard worked as a domestic servant'.[38]

As with the male patients, not all women can easily be categorized as paupers, or even assumed to be from the working class. Joseph Melling identified one particularly ambiguous group, governesses, who, he pointed out, were often recruited from families of a good social status, frequently linked to professional backgrounds.[39] Although there were considerably less governesses than domestic servants in England and Wales, they too were vulnerable, as their accommodation was invariably tied to their employment. Governesses were a sensitive issue; they had to be 'well-bred' so as to be fit for instilling the correct virtues into the children of the middle and upper classes. Thus they were essentially of the same class but usually isolated within the household. The difficulty was that the middle classes were used to dealing with their servants but had no experience of dealing with their own kind.[40] No governesses were admitted to Brookwood in 1871 and 1881, but in 1884 there were six and a further seven in 1891. At Holloway, most female patients were recorded as not having an occupation. Occasionally governesses were admitted, but they could also be recorded as nurses, teachers or as 'companions'.

Most patients admitted to Holloway were unmarried; in 1890, for example, 65 per cent were single, of whom nearly three-quarters were women. Rees Philipps observed that, among the single and widowed patients admitted in 1892, 'the female sex preponderated to the extent of forty-five and fifty-five per cent respectively'.[41] A sample of 1,003 certified and voluntary female patients admitted from 1895 to 1905 verifies this and shows that 64 per cent were single (including widows). Amongst the voluntary patients, the figure is 71 per cent, suggesting that some of these unmarried women, or their families, may have seen the sanatorium as an attractive residential option. This had repercussions for the recovery rates and the dominance of women as residual patients.[42]

According to the 1891 census, there were nearly one million more women than men in England and Wales.[43] The latter half of the nineteenth century had

seen the rise of the culture of the single man, as it became more socially acceptable for middle-class men to delay marriage in order to focus on establishing
their fortune, if they married at all.[44] Many more men's clubs opened, such as
the luxury Albany 'men only' accommodation in Piccadilly, London, which
offered comfort and male companionship. Prostitution was rife. Not only were
there fewer men, but seemingly fewer reasons for them to marry. Despite the
emergence of employment and education opportunities, middle-class women's
perceived and ultimate destiny remained marriage. As John Tosh has pointed out,
for better-off families who employed servants, there were fewer domestic duties
to occupy unmarried women, and, for those from the lower income brackets, no
option of a life-long income.[45] Unmarried women may have felt marginalized,
lonely, frustrated and unfulfilled, which possibly led to some psychotic behavioural patterns, or, they simply became a burden to their families. This may have
affected the numbers admitted to Holloway as the women themselves, and their
relatives, chose this prestigious establishment as being suitable for their refuge
or containment. Reflecting social mores and the status quo, it is unsurprising
that it was predominantly the male family members, fathers, bothers, adult sons
and brothers-in-law, who petitioned for the certification and incarceration of
the women who attended the Holloway Sanatorium. As previously stated, the
data does not support Showalter's allegation of disproportionate incarceration
of women in the nineteenth century.

The single women admitted to Holloway tended to be younger than at
Brookwood; nearly two-thirds were under the age of forty-five, and so of
childbearing age, but with no socially acceptable outlets for sexual feelings and
limited intellectual opportunities or acceptable areas of employment. Charlotte
MacKenzie found evidence that the insanity of some of the female patients at
Ticehurst had initially been detected by families and doctors when the patient
had sought advice with regard to gynaecological problems; whilst it is feasible
that this may have been the case at Holloway, there is no hard evidence of this.[46]

It is not possible to decipher particular patterns for the incarceration of married women in Holloway, nor is it possible to determine consistent behavioural
criteria that would have led their relatives to have them certified and submitted
to medical scrutiny. However, some types of personal behaviour were deemed
inappropriate for married women, and allegedly caused distress to their husbands and families. According to the evidence presented by their husbands,
and other (often) male relatives that was recorded in the certificates of insanity,
many women were described as having exhibited various forms of 'erotic' behaviour or inappropriate conduct whilst in public. The evidence provided by Mary
Emmaline's husband was not untypical. He informed the doctor that his wife's
conversation was 'improper and even coarse in the presence of her children'.[47] He
also testified that 'She has frequently made her escape from the house at night

and without proper clothes' and further, 'She shows entire incapacity for managing her house and looking after herself'.[48] Husbands' concerns regarding the
behaviour of their wives were not limited to the women admitted to Holloway.
Georgina F., a Brookwood patient, came from a more affluent background and
had been living abroad in Ceylon with her husband, when in 1897, she suffered
from an attack of malarial fever which was identified as the cause of her subsequent mental instability. She was returned to England and was treated in both
Cardiff and Kingston infirmaries prior to being admitted to Brookwood, where
she slowly improved. Her possible discharge came up for review in April 1906,
but her husband reacted badly to this news. He expressed his anxiety about her
unreasonable behaviour, particularly during her menstrual cycle when, in his
opinion, her personal conduct became unacceptable in a wife and mother. He
informed the superintendent:

> Although she has improved in her detention at Brookwood, I respectfully request
> that her cure may be permanent before discharged as the conditions of living with
> her, especially when she is passing through her monthly periods, are, for me practi-
> cally intolerable, her disease taking the form of excessive obstinacy & hatred towards
> our child aged 10 years & myself & refusal to allow anyone else in the house or with
> her. The mother's conduct during these attacks have an effect upon the nervous sys-
> tem of the child, which has now lately begun to improve.[49]

At both Brookwood and Holloway, attempted suicide or violence directed at
self or others was often the catalyst that caused families to seek professional and
institutional care. This desire to keep themselves and their relative safe transcended the age, sex or status of the patient. Jeanie W. was brought to Holloway
by her mother in November 1894 following her self-attempted hanging at her
family home in Chelsea. Four days after her admission, she tried self-strangulation with tape, although this attempt was described in her notes as being 'half
hearted'. This was her only serious transgression during her one year stay as a certified patient; she then went on to spend a further month as a voluntary boarder
before she returned to her family.[50]

Six per cent of male admissions to Holloway were widowers. Altogether,
three-quarters of the men admitted to Holloway in the period 1885–8 were single and were similar to the single women in being, on average, younger than their
married counterparts. This differs from the findings at the private establishment
of Wonford House, where almost half the male patients were married.[51] Whilst
the model of the family prepared to spend in order to cure the breadwinner has
been discussed (see above), the high numbers of single middle-class males admitted to Holloway indicates that it may have been the income-earning potential
of all males that deemed them worthy of the investment in medical treatment.

By the early 1890s, however, there was a small but perceptible shift and slightly more married men were being admitted for care.

Concerned women also brought their male relatives to the sanatorium for treatment, such as the wife of George C. in 1891. She described her husband as being restless and excitable; he kept her awake by walking around the house throughout the night, and he was 'peculiar in many respects'.[52] He was sixty-five, a retired servant (thus not conventionally middle-class), but was seen by his family as being worth the financial outlay to be treated at Holloway. He lived only for another three years before he died of GPI. Although wives and mothers played their part in the incarceration process, most men were brought to the attention of the authorities by their male relatives, in keeping with societal conventions. Robert C. was a surgeon who was brought to Holloway in April 1892 by his father and brother, who were also surgeons.[53] Robert was single, aged thirty-six and was suffering from delusions and depression. His relatives were unable to cope with his ramblings and incoherence, his excessive shopping sprees and hoarding of food in his bedroom. Although his strange behaviour was clearly troubling (he also would pretend to be deaf and dumb), it is likely that his male relatives' sensibilities were heightened by the fact that Robert's mother had been certified insane some years previously.[54] However, other records show that Robert's family remained supportive towards him for the remainder of his life.

With regard to the occupational status of the patients admitted to Holloway, it is only possible to make some summary observations due to the paucity of recorded information. The 1886 sanatorium rules and regulations stated that no patient or boarder was to be admitted to Holloway, 'unless in the opinion of the House Committee, she or he has held such a respectable position in society as unfits him or her for association with paupers'.[55] The admission registers endorse this requirement as most patients were of independent means, or there was no recorded occupation. There were also patients who were upper class, titled or landed gentry, although defining 'middle-class' must have presented some problems for the asylum's management. The management had anticipated that their typical patients would include students, barristers or clergymen and those 'whose minds are filled with illusions on account of domestic troubles or bereavements'.[56] Such men were represented together with officers from the armed forces, solicitors, medical men, accountants, farmers, artists and actors, clerks from a variety of sectors, merchants and commodities dealers. But nearly a third (32 per cent) of men was described as having no occupation or being of independent means. The registers also reveal a few atypical admissions, such as servants and commercial travellers. Most female patients were of independent means or were gentlewomen; for example, in 1894, 85 per cent of the women admitted had no given occupation and were mostly described as being 'of good social standing'. Collating this information for the sanatorium's management was important: 'In regulating admissions we have to see that in social standing the patients are those for whom the Hospital is intended'.[57] It was also important for the sanatorium to attempt to balance the class and fee-paying abilities of their patients.

Voluntary Boarders

One unique group of patients at Holloway was the voluntary boarders (see Figure 4.5). Comprehensive records were not maintained for these patients so there are many instances of missing information and data, and occasionally even basic admission data was not documented.[58]

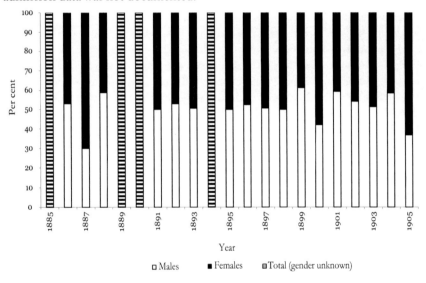

Figure 4.5: Holloway Sanatorium, general patient admissions by sex, 1885–1905, voluntary boarders. Source: Holloway Admission Registers and Annual Reports, Surrey History Centre.

Admitting a sizeable number of uncertified patients to the Holloway Sanatorium was part of a therapeutic strategy that was much favoured by the management. Occasionally its use brought them into dispute with the Commissioners in Lunacy, especially before the 1890 Lunacy Act, which recognized registered hospitals' practice of admitting non-certified patients.[59] In 1890, voluntary admissions (or 'boarders') accounted for nearly 35 per cent of all new patients. This was not an unusual proportion. Of these boarders, nearly a quarter were certified and transferred to the patients' list, usually within the course of the first few days. During the first 23 years of operation (1885–1905), a total of 2,815 certified patients, together with 1,258 voluntary boarders, were treated at the sanatorium. Just like other patients, boarders were also entitled to apply for charitable assistance and could be admitted for treatment on this basis.

The medical staff strongly believed that the voluntary admission procedure not only mitigated the trauma of admission but positively assisted the recovery process. The patient was arguably more relaxed, and during that period of time, the staff's observations could lead to a more accurate diagnosis. But there was a consensus amongst the management that this group of patients could be particularly demanding. This was especially so if they remained voluntary boarders for a lengthy period of time; they behaved like hotel guests, often failed to observe hospital regulations or refused treatment. However, their status could change and they could be certified if the doctors judged a patient to be in need of compulsory treatment. A reception order would be duly issued, and the patients' medical details transferred from the voluntary (and less regimented) case books to the 'patients' list', all within a matter of days. There were exceptions, and some patients were never certified, even if they were readmitted on several occasions.

The sanatorium's management estimated that approximately one-third of the boarders 'drift[ed] into certifiable insanity'.[60] The superintendent robustly defended Holloway's procedures against accusations of commercial opportunism. He pointed out that, to the contrary, if certification became necessary, a transfer to another hospital was usually the first recommendation so that the patient did not bear any resentment towards the sanatorium. Patient status within the sanatorium could fluctuate; they may have become certified patients (and later revert back to voluntary status) in what appears to have been a very flexible system. Eva Margaret was typical. She was twenty-one years of age when she was first brought to the sanatorium in 1898 by her mother as a voluntary boarder. She suffered from mania, and over the next eight years returned to Holloway many times as both certified patient and voluntary boarder.[61] She was eventually discharged as 'not improved' to the Coppice, Nottingham.[62]

For some voluntary patients, the sanatorium became a safe haven and once 'recovered', some of these patients chose to remain there as boarders. Several were middle-aged women, such as 47-year-old unmarried former schoolmistress, Mary Ann, who had plagued the medical superintendent with her declarations of love throughout her stay. Laundry work, not something she would have been familiar with, reportedly relieved her 'erotic' disposition, and, having nowhere else to go, she elected to stay at Holloway for many more years.[63] Readmissions and prolonged periods of residence were slightly more evident amongst Holloway's voluntary boarders than the certified patients. This does not necessarily suggest families conspired against female family members but rather that there was a perceived lack of options for some following discharge.

The voluntary patients brought tangible benefits to the sanatorium; they offered the potential for additional income, and allowed those with less serious conditions (such as mild epilepsy) to be admitted for respite care. As already noted, Holloway's management was obliged to admit several higher-class patients in order to offset the fees of charitable cases. This may also indicate the trend for charitable asylums to increase their percentage of high payers and thus assume more of an upper-class profile, a practice seen at both Bethlem and Ticehurst.[64] The Chancery lunatics who were admitted had a guaranteed income from the trustees of their estates, so they were likely to have been welcomed on financial grounds. There were relatively few of these patients at Holloway, unlike at Ticehurst, where (by 1875) they not only paid the highest fees, but accounted for nearly one-quarter of the patients.[65]

Outcomes

At Brookwood, typically, patients were either discharged as recovered within less than a year, or else they became long-term inmates. The most likely outcomes were discharge (including 'relieved' or 'not improved'), or death. In 1892, for example, thirty-six patients had been 'under treatment' for less than six months, twenty-seven for six to nine months, and seven for between nine and twelve months. By way of exception, one woman who was discharged as recovered had spent twenty-five years as a Brookwood patient.[66] This endorses earlier findings by Ray whose sampling of patients in the 1870s and 1890s showed high admission rates but also indicated a relatively high turnover; 47 per cent (1870s) and 54 per cent (1890s) of cases were 'resolved' in either of these ways.[67]

Each year, many inmates were discharged as 'relieved' or 'not improved'; these somewhat ambiguous terms were applied to patients who were either taken into care by friends or transferred to other asylums. But many of the discharged patients were not considered sufficiently well and the asylum's relatively poor recovery record acknowledged by the management and reported by other agencies, such as the Commissioners in Lunacy, was an ongoing concern. In his study, Ray has suggested that medical superintendents exhibited a preoccupation with patient chronicity in the late nineteenth century, which, he alleges, was not so much a response to the overcrowding of the asylums, but rather was an indication that insanity was increasingly seen as a 'permanent impairment'.[68] The Brookwood records indicate that this may have been the case in that the later annual reports increasingly focus on patients' poor (mental) condition and the influence of possible hereditary factors. In 1892, with a daily average number of 1,086 patients (the highest since opening), the second superintendent, Dr Barton, reported that recoveries (as a proportion of the admissions) accounted for only 31 per cent (n. 82) and that this was nearly 11 per cent lower than the previous year which he believed was due to 'the unfavourable character of the admissions'.[69] Five years later, in 1897, the disastrous recovery rate of 28.57 per cent was once more blamed on the 'highly unfavourable character of the admissions'.[70] However, pessimism was alleviated by occasional successes; in 1900, Dr Barton was pleased to report that the year 1899 had seen the highest recovery rate for ten years, namely 45.16 per cent.[71]

Brookwood's death rates were relatively high, sometimes accounting for 15 per cent of admissions, and together with the low recovery rates, especially amongst young inmates, could be considered as indicative of the failures of the asylum's therapeutic regime. This was not helped by various environmental problems such as overcrowding, inadequate water and insufficient air supply in the wards, particularly during the earlier years. However, it should be remembered that the asylum's high intake of physically weak and chronic patients had the strongest impact on the figures. Contagious diseases spread quickly, and the poor physical condition of some patients hindered their treatment. As the medical superintendent and his staff regarded many such patients as incurable, it is possible that a minimalist care regime was provided for these patients. Between 1865 and 1896, one-third of Brookwood inmates died in the asylum, a not dissimilar figure to that seen at Devon County Asylum.[72] More men died than women, many as a result of GPI.

Women may not have been overly represented amongst admissions to Brookwood but they were the largest proportion of patients who remained in the asylum at the end of each year, a pattern replicated at Holloway. Melling has pointed out that a strong belief was emerging that long periods of incarceration were essential for all patients, regardless of their sex, and that this accorded with theories of inherent insanity and feeblemindedness.[73] There is evidence of an increased emphasis on hereditary factors in insanity but this does not affect the key findings here for the period under study.

At Brookwood, from 1867 to 1896 (see Figure 4.6), women accounted for an average of 58 per cent of the patients. This meant that in some years there were as many as two hundred more women than men still incarcerated at the end of the year.[74] At Denbigh Asylum, Pamela Michael has also observed that women tended to stay longer than men.[75] Women's natural longevity has already been cited as a contributory factor but some women also benefited from regular meals, as well as the respite from childbearing and other familial duties, and often physically improved during their stay.[76] Many women enjoyed a substantially better diet than outside as men's low or irregular wages often made it difficult for them to adequately support their families. As a result, many married women went without sufficient food and consequently suffered worse health than married men.[77] The regular meals and the 'extras' that were given to particularly feeble patients, it has been suggested, were particularly relevant in cases of puerperal insanity, where women were allowed the time and space to recover physically and mentally from childbirth.[78]

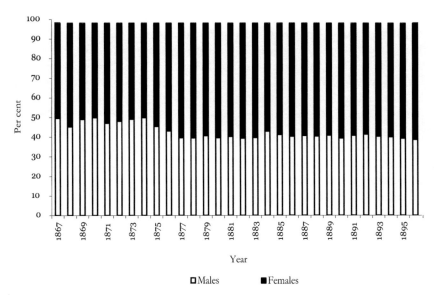

Figure 4.6: Brookwood Asylum, patients remaining by sex, 1867–96. Source: Patient Admissions Registers, Surrey History Centre.

Brookwood's high rates of long-stay female inmates are partially explained by the higher death rates amongst male patients, a fact that was highlighted by the medical superintendent in his 1871 report. Also, male admissions across the country occasionally outnumbered that of females, as, according to the superintendent, they were more prone to 'mental impairment'.[79] This view suggests contemporary empathy with the many pressures that men were subjected to, such as physical work, intellectual pursuits and providing for families. Arguably, this perspective could be substantiated by the higher rates of completed male suicides (discussed in more detail in Chapter 6). The superintendent pointed out in his reports the regularly higher male mortality rates in the asylum.[80] Many men at Brookwood were diagnosed as suffering from GPI. In 1869, it accounted for 22 per cent of all the male deaths in Brookwood and this figure increased steadily.[81] In 1875, forty-four men died of this disease as opposed to twenty-seven women. Until 1890, GPI was held to be responsible for over 33 per cent of all male deaths and up to 24 per cent of females at Brookwood.[82]

It is arguable that working-class women were less financially independent, more likely to become impoverished if orphaned, deserted or unemployed, and that these factors were reasons for their remaining in the asylum. In addition, the stigma of being a discharged lunatic would have further hindered their employment opportunities which under normal circumstances were more limited than men's. Women's earning potential was only between one-third and one-half of that of male manual workers.[83] As the century drew to a close, attempts to reduce the numbers of outdoor paupers had been particularly successful with regard to women in need. This was not achieved by increased prosperity but rather by principally cutting the outdoor relief previously granted to wives of able-bodied men, single childless women, and the wives of prisoners and service men, although there was also a decline in support for widows.[84] The 1899 Brookwood annual report revealed that ninety-eight males, but only sixty-eight females, were discharged that year, and that, whilst previously, variations in the mortality rate may have been a contributing factor, by this time the overall death rate was equal among the sexes. This suggests a lack of support for newly discharged women as well as hereditary fears gaining momentum.

Predictably, some patients attempted to escape from Brookwood, behaviour that was deemed symptomatic of mental instability and treated accordingly. Henry A., brought from his home to Brookwood in June 1871, exhibited violent and suicidal behaviour and was treated with a shower bath to calm him down. However, after one such occasion, he broke a window on the second floor, dropped to the ground and ran across the grounds before being detained near the chapel. He was given a purgative 'with a view to occupy him, and divert his mind'. Undeterred, he made six further escape attempts over the next three months, none of which gained him more than a few hours of freedom.[85] Attempted escapes were reported most years; in 1898 for example, there were eight, only one of which was ultimately successful. Having taken advantage of the relative freedom enjoyed by working in a gang of gardening patients, this particular male patient seized his opportunity to scale the boundary fence on the Guildford Road. He was not recaptured, and after the statutory fourteen-day period had expired, his name was removed from the asylum records.[86]

At Holloway, the recovery rate initially did not differ vastly from that at Brookwood; for example, in 1887 it stood at 33.3 per cent for certified patients of both sexes, although this rate would have been higher if the voluntary patients had been included.[87] However, death rates were lower during the early years; in 1887 for example, they stood at 7.3 per cent, which the superintendent still felt was too high. He attributed this to having admitted too many weak and feeble patients to the sanatorium, thus echoing the same concerns as his counterpart at Brookwood.[88] By 1895, however, Holloway's management was recording improved rates that served to emphasize the differences between the private and public system; the recovery rate (on admissions and excluding transfers) stood at 65 per cent, with a death rate of just under 4 per cent.[89] The same year at Brookwood, recoveries stood at nearly 32 per cent with a death rate of 12.5 per cent.[90]

At Holloway Sanatorium, women stayed longer than men and they were frequently readmitted, both practices which directly contradicted the founding rules:

no patient will be allowed to remain an inmate of the institution for a longer period than twelve months; no patient will be received whose case is considered hopeless; no patient will be allowed to enter the sanatorium after having been discharged.[91]

Just as at Brookwood, more women than men were residual patients at the end of each year, accounting for more than 60 per cent (1885–8) and 58 per cent in 1895, the only years for which this data is available at Holloway. Most of these long-term female inmates were either unmarried or widowed.[92]

In 1887, women accounted for 70 per cent of the voluntary boarders who were admitted, and for 75 per cent of those voluntary patients who remained at the end of the year.[93] As above, the higher number of residual female patients is explained partially by social restrictions and few opportunities. Widowed or unmarried middle-class women were perhaps less likely than working-class women to be found a useful position within the family structure. For many male and female voluntary patients, it was sometimes their choice to remain at the sanatorium. This was not unwelcome; as Dr Moore (the successor to Rees Philipps) observed: 'Most of the voluntary boarders at present in residence have been patients who, on recovery, preferred to remain here. I find them useful in many ways, and they take a prominent part in the social life of the Hospital.'[94]

Class transcended some factors; just as at Brookwood, female longevity and higher male mortality within the sanatorium contributed to the larger number of women remaining at the end of the year. Similarly, many men admitted to Holloway were diagnosed as general paralytics (suffering from tertiary syphilis). At Holloway, this disease accounted for the death of three out of every four men.[95] Death rates for the sanatorium hovered between 7 and 9 per cent, and the higher male death rates were astonishingly ascribed by the superintendent to 'the almost complete immunity from general paralysis enjoyed by the female sex'.[96]

Holloway patients who were discharged as 'relieved' or 'not improved' were either transferred to other private institutions or returned home to their families. Just as at Brookwood, some families were reluctant to receive their relatives back into the fold; the superintendent noted a case where a female patient was not wanted home despite the fact that she was no longer insane: 'One lady, whose friends were unwilling to remove her, was discharged relieved, by order of the Commissioners in Lunacy, who, after an interview with her, thought that she was able to take care of herself'.[97] There were similar instances of family 'rejection' at Brookwood as seen above, and such unwillingness, while often difficult to interpret, may have been motivated by feelings of repugnance or ineptitude.

Despite the luxurious surroundings, patients did not always wish to stay at Holloway and also attempted to escape, although a few of these efforts were described by the management as being 'more in the nature of wandering from home'. This was the view adopted when patients were found drinking in the local inn, for example, or if they were recaptured whilst attending some prestigious social event. Some did return to the sanatorium of their own accord, as reported in 1896 when two out of three escapees that year did so.[98]

Conclusion

The research into the patients at Brookwood Asylum and Holloway Sanatorium has challenged the assumption that women were disproportionately incarcerated in the nineteenth century. The ratio of male-to-female patients admitted was roughly comparable to that of other lunatic asylums and in the general population. Brookwood received a high percentage of patients from the workhouses, many of whom were young men who were often physically as well as mentally ill. Despite the management's frustration at the Poor Law union policy that had led to their transferal to the asylum, they tried to provide the best possible care and safety for these patients. Brookwood's patients' previous occupations demonstrate that, although this was a Poor Law institution, patients had been employed before their initial admission to the workhouse, and that the range of occupations span the spectrum, including the professions. At Holloway, fewer occupations were represented, with the majority being 'gentlemen' of independent means. The working history of female patients (particularly at Brookwood) is likely to have been under-recorded. Single and widowed patients were more likely to be admitted to both asylums, and Holloway's female patients were predominantly middle-aged.

In many respects, Brookwood patients' experience reflects that outlined by historians such as Wright in his work on Bucks County Asylum, Stone. As Wright has pointed out, asylum incarceration for most patients was a temporary experience, with between 40 and 60 per cent of patients in county asylums staying for twelve months or less.[99] In 1981, Laurence Ray's work on pauper patients in Brookwood and Lancaster Asylum noted that the long-term confinement of patients was exceptional.[100] Yet still the image of the long-term patient has persisted and was utilized by some historians, such as Showalter, to suggest that women in particular suffered discrimination and resultant over-admission to asylums. This is not supported by the data examined here, which shows only marginally more women than men were admitted to both asylums over the period. If they did not recover to be discharged quickly, however, they were likely to be incarcerated for long periods of time, so that women did form the majority of remaining patients in both Brookwood and Holloway at the end of each year. It might be argued that women were not admitted in greater numbers, but, rather, that they had limited options as to where they might be discharged to, particularly once removed from the family environment.

Holloway's environment was arguably attractive to unmarried women with limited career and personal options, as well as for single men and the widowed. Their incarceration potentially eased the family's burden, particularly if the patient was eccentric, difficult or had some physical or mental debility that placed strains on the family unit. Not all Holloway's patients were 'middle class'; many upper-class patients who paid the top rate of fees were admitted. There was also the sanatorium's involvement with the After-Care Association which allowed for recuperating lunatics of all classes to be cared for within the sanatorium environment, which further indicates the fluid interpretation of this term. Voluntary admissions to Holloway added dimension to the profile of Holloway's patients, in that these patients caused supervisory problems, and brought the institution into conflict with the Commissioners in Lunacy.

5 THE TAXONOMY AND TREATMENT OF INSANITY

Introduction

In their respective published annual reports, the management of both asylums recorded the recovery rates and deaths of their patients as these provided tangible evidence of the effectiveness of the asylums' therapeutic regime. Many reasons were offered to explain disappointing results. The huge numbers of admissions to county asylums in the nineteenth century placed a considerable administrative and financial burden on these institutions. In previous chapters, it has been shown that at Brookwood the management was initially unprepared for the huge demand for places from the county's workhouses, and that some workhouse patients arrived in appalling physical and mental condition. The result was a 'residual' asylum population, which has led to the suggestion that any 'curative ideals' were restricted to the early years of the nineteenth century when the medical superintendents had the time to experiment with a variety of therapeutics.[1] This argument, however, simplifies the later nineteenth-century asylum therapeutic response and minimizes the continued efforts made by doctors to restore their patients to 'normality' within financial and practical constraints. Melling and Forsythe argue that statistics – i.e. patient admissions, length of stay and reason for discharge – provide recovery rates that may assist an understanding of the impact of treatment.[2] On the assumption that one of the primary aims of the nineteenth-century asylum was to cure its patients, one might agree with the management boards of both institutions, that recovery and death rates were reasonable indicators of success. The Commissioners in Lunacy certainly required this information from public asylums, and the private sector asylums also carefully monitored their recovery and death rates. In part, this was done to measure their effectiveness against competitors and thus attract fee-paying patients.

The moral, physical and chemical therapies used at Brookwood and Holloway will be examined here. In general terms, asylums embraced what was termed 'moral therapy'. Within institutional care, this encompassed the entire asylum

environment and regime, with every detail and component of daily life contributing to therapeutic efficacy. 'Moral therapy', as Wright has pointed out, was
originally a lay initiative that was quickly co-opted by the emergent specialists
in psychological medicine, particularly the medical superintendents of the new
county pauper asylums.[3] Strongly associated with the York Retreat, moral treatment emphasized a more humane approach to caring for the insane that rejected
physical restraint, but that did require patient co-operation. Ray has described
this method of treatment as being most appropriate for what he terms the 'sick-
role construction [that] views madness as a transitory condition' that decreed
that the condition was primarily caused by external factors such as poverty,
stress, emotional problems or 'inadequate moral education'.[4] Thus, the removal
of a patient from a stressful or damaging environment to an asylum could only
be beneficial, while providing the opportunity for him/her to regain control of
emotions and to self-regulate behaviour.

As admissions to asylums increased, and recovery rates appeared to stagnate,
there were calls for more scientific research into mental illness, and revisions of
medical methodology to reflect the more humane approach to incarcerating the
insane. The so-called psychiatric approach, which viewed insanity as resulting
from 'brain pathology', overlapped with principles of moral treatment, but the
two were not entirely contradictory and did not necessarily imply an unfavourable outcome. At the same time, theories regarding hereditary causes of insanity
were emerging, and these gradually assumed more prominence.[5] Hereditary
causes were strongly associated with poor prognosis, yet Samuel Tuke cautioned
against adopting this essentially pessimistic view.[6] As Ray has pointed out, this
warning went largely unheeded, and caution in linking hereditary with constitu-
tional causes declined by the second half of the nineteenth century. The impact
of what he refers to as the 'impaired identity' model was most clearly articulated
by Henry Maudsley who believed that unchecked insanity was passed down the
generations and ultimately ended in the most extreme condition of idiocy.[7]

Scull's work examined how rapid institutional growth restricted the proper
implementation of moral treatment, diluted the therapeutic role of the superintendent, and created difficulties in adhering to policies of non-restraint.[8] This
might suggest that the therapeutic regime failed, but the turnover of patients at
Brookwood and the relative successes, as discussed in previous chapters, show
that this was not always the case. Brookwood embraced the principles of moral
therapy and was admired by contemporaries for this. Despite burgeoning numbers, the medical staff took advantage of whatever tools were available to treat
patients whom they believed had some chance of recovery. That is not to say that
punitive measures were never adopted, but that they were rarely used. Arguably,
seclusion required some coercion, but this option, which was used for violent

or difficult patients, was interpreted and applied in a humane fashion by Brookwood's first medical superintendents.[9]

As Digby found at the York Retreat, the value of specific therapeutic treatments can be difficult to assess. One possible approach is to consider the extent of medical assessment, and the changing nature of medical remedies administered to the patients, although scant evidence makes conclusions necessarily tentative.[10] With regular inspections by the Commissioners in Lunacy, asylums were obliged to conform to many bureaucratic practices, as well as maintain detailed records and medical case books in order to clearly record the details of each patient's individual case and subsequent treatment. As no specific record of the drugs that were administered has survived, it has been necessary to consider those records where there are references to physical and chemical treatments. However, recording in case books was often erratic, and with long-term cases, note-taking invariably deteriorated into rudimentary entries; in this way, they also represented collaboration between the medical staff who were in broad agreement as to the unlikelihood of some patients ever improving. Staff often recorded quite subjective views on their patients and provided evidence as to the difficulties they experienced whilst trying to maintain an orderly therapeutic environment.[11]

Chemical or physical treatments were usually reserved for the most difficult cases, such as those who suffered from bouts of mania, general paralysis of the insane, or who were violent or suicidal. At Brookwood, the volume of patients and financial constraints influenced who was selected for chemical treatment, and for how long. Case books indicate that medication was discontinued if an improvement was not apparent within a relatively short space of time. In this age of non-restraint, blisters, dry-packs, shower baths and seclusion were used at both asylums, suggesting that an eclectic mixture of treatments were employed. There is also evidence of surgery being carried out at Brookwood in an attempt to elicit a cure; this was a relatively unusual procedure in a public asylum, and one which aroused considerable medical interest.[12]

At Holloway, the case books and annual reports suggest that there was a broader range of chemical and physical treatments available, including early electric therapy. Many of these were innovative at the time and necessitated training staff in new procedures, such as massage and gym exercise. An incomplete drug manual has survived (discussed below), which provides some insight into the most commonly used medicines. The impression at Holloway is that, due to fewer financial restrictions, there was a much more routine application of medicinal treatment in order to relieve both mental and physical symptoms. This disregard for cost, and the use of cutting-edge treatment, would have also been the expectation of many patients and their families.

Diagnosis

The therapeutic regime began with admission and diagnosis. Diagnosis was not standardized and was influenced by class and gender perceptions as well as the evidence presented by friends and relatives of the patient. This was an imperfect system, and as G. E. Berrious has detailed extensively, the definitions of terms such as mania and melancholia have changed over time.[13] The classification of two patients with allegedly the same illness did not depend on them exhibiting the same symptoms. Details of the patient's social and medical history were recorded during the admission process, together with evidence taken from official sources as well as from the patient's family and friends. The patient's physical characteristics were noted, along with an assessment of his/her current mental condition and any known suicidal or violent tendencies. Health and general bodily descriptions were also included, and these were not always entirely objective.

The patients at Brookwood and Holloway suffered primarily from the same diseases; limited scientific research at this time meant a restricted medical vocabulary and patients were broadly assessed according to the same criteria, often based on social evaluations. The primary illnesses were dementia; mania and melancholia, acute or chronic; sometimes accompanied by additional complications such as suicidal or dangerous behaviour or epileptic attacks. The information used here refers to the diagnosis of the patient at the time of admission, as this was consistently recorded and therefore measurable. There was some contemporary recognition of the inherent difficulties of the diagnostic terms: 'Mania, melancholia, and dementia are merely convenient clinical terms to express the mental condition of a patient at a given time, and have no higher function'.[14]

The initial diagnosis could alter during the patient's stay; for example, some long-term patients might develop symptoms of dementia, or their mania might subside. Conditions such as epilepsy and GPI, which required intensive nursing care, were commonly identified in patients at both asylums. As noted by Berrios, GPI was often attributed to patients with depression who went on to develop dementia.[15]

Evidence from the certificates of insanity and case books of both asylums indicate that similar diagnostic criteria were applied to both men and women, although these were influenced to an extent by an expectation as to what was appropriate and socially acceptable behaviour for either sex.[16] Certain types of insanity were more likely to be identified with one particular sex. For example, mania, GPI and idiocy were most usually diagnosed and associated with males, and what Wright has referred to as 'mood disorders' such as melancholia or mania with depression (and of course puerperal insanity) were associated with female patients.[17] The initial diagnosis was predominantly based on the certificates of insanity that accompanied the patients' admission. These contained a significant amount of lay evidence which was often vague and thus open to interpretation. As noted, the original diagnosis could be altered if additional or different symptoms emerged whilst the patient was under surveillance during their stay. Conversely, some alleged indications of insanity were never witnessed once the patient was in the asylum.[18]

Diagnosis, undertaken as soon as possible following admission, should not be confused with classification. Arguably, classification was basic and could be utilized to assist patient management. Whilst it did not necessarily mean a total eradication of individuality, generalizations occurred that could only be rectified by maintaining a focus on the individual, as opposed to the many.[19] However, the value of classification or identification of the patient's ailment was that it could be used as a way of ensuring the correct therapeutic approach which might lead to recovery. Early attempts were rudimentary; for example, convalescents were separated from incurables, and the noisy from the quiet. These relatively crude categorizations became more refined over time and were deemed largely beneficial, as seen when separation formed the basis for the implementation of Tuke's practices at York. He did not believe in large numbers of patients being herded together, but rather he attempted to organize them into small supportive groups – 'little families' – and proposed classification according to the extent of the disease rather than the diagnosis itself.[20] This was later replicated in many other asylums. At Brookwood, staff cottages were utilized as smaller, more relaxed units where trusted patients lived; twelve were regularly lodged with the farm bailiff, for example. This practice was also seen at Holloway but was not restricted to manageable patients; violent and difficult male patients were cared for in their own specialized unit in the grounds known as The Retreat, where they formed their own highly secure community.

Rees Philipps thought it was impossible to have too much subdivision and classification of the patients, and that:

> No convalescent patient, no newly admitted one with any powers of observation left, should ever be frightened by the sight or sound of a noisy, violent, or obscene lunatic. In the ideal asylum the divisions made should be made many and diverse in their style and fittings; villas, cottage homes, a seaside branch, a town house if the asylum is in the country, farmhouse accommodation, all should be provided, and all would tend to promote the comfort and cure of the patients.[21]

Disease and Causes

Dementia

Figures 5.1a and 5.1b illustrate the prevelance of dementia, by age and sex, amongst the patients, as diagnosed on admission.[22]

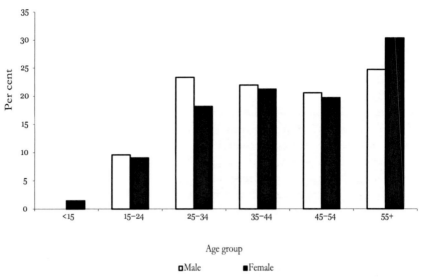

Figure 5.1a: Admissions to Brookwood Asylum by disease: dementia (N = 134).

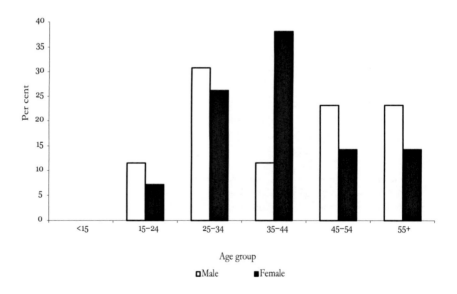

Figure 5.1b: Admissions to Holloway Sanatorium by disease: dementia (N = 68).

At Brookwood, dementia was attributed to 15 per cent of males and 21 per cent of females. When considering the Brookwood admissions data for three selected years (1871, 1881 and 1891), the graphs show that dementia was more commonly diagnosed in older men and women; it accounted for nearly 30 per cent of women over fifty-five years of age. The Holloway data shows that women in the 35–44 year age group were the main group diagnosed as suffering from this disease, nearly three times more than men of the same age. In a sample for 1888, dementia accounted for 15 per cent of the admissions; these patients were less likely to recover and no sufferers were discharged that year.[23] In long-term patients the diagnosis often altered over the years; dementia could be detected in both maniacal and melancholic patients of either sex and it was often associated with the latter stages of GPI. As Melling and Forsyth have stated, the medical diagnoses of the insane were 'less precise and rigorous than we might have expected'.[24]

Mania

Figures 5.2a and 5.2b look at the percentage of patients diagnosed with mania upon admission to the two asylums, again by age and sex, with the data extrapolated from the same sources as before.

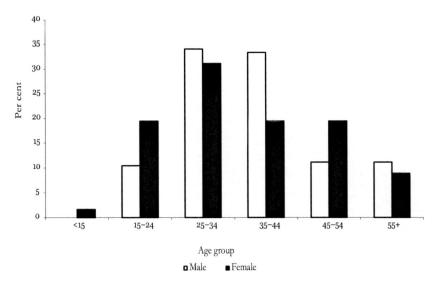

Figure 5.2a: Admissions to Brookwood Asylum by disease: mania (N = 324).

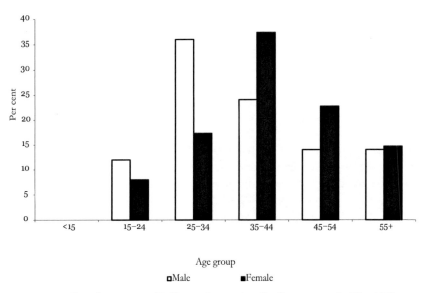

Age group

□Male   ■Female

Figure 5.2b: Admissions to Holloway Sanatorium by disease: mania (N = 125).

Nearly half of all male and female patients admitted to Brookwood were diagnosed with mania, particularly the 25–44 year age groups. Mania was prevalent in men and, as shown, it was the males aged 35–44 years who accounted for 30 per cent of all maniacal admissions to the asylum. At Holloway, it was a different picture; men aged 25–34 years only, were more than twice as likely as women of the same age to suffer from mania (34 per cent as opposed to 15 per cent). Women aged 35–44 years accounted for over 35 per cent of mania admissions (as opposed to less than 20 per cent at Brookwood) and women dominated the other remaining age groups. Taking the admissions for 1888 as an example, 41 per cent suffered from acute or chronic mania, and patients with this illness accounted for 28 per cent of the year's discharges.

Melancholia

Figures 5.3a and 5.3b show the percentage of new patients diagnosed as suffering from melancholia on admission to Brookwood and Holloway. Again, it is not possible to know how many patients may have developed symptoms of melancholia later during their stay.

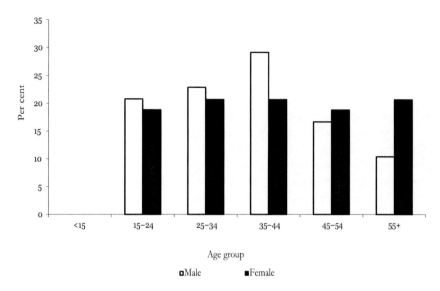

Figure 5.3a: Admissions to Brookwood Asylum by disease: melancholia (N = 101). Data extrapolated from the Admissions Registers for Brookwood and Holloway, held at SHC.

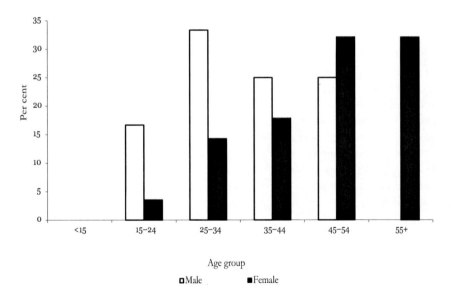

Figure 5.3b: Admissions to Holloway Sanatorium by disease: melancholia (N = 40). Data extrapolated from the Admissions Registers for Brookwood and Holloway, held at SHC.

Melancholia accounted for nearly a third of all admissions to Brookwood and was evenly distributed between men and women across all age groups, although it was slightly more prevalent in men under the age of forty-four. This was also the case at Holloway. Melancholia was a common diagnosis for women over forty-four years (nearly a third of patients) being admitted to Holloway. For example, in 1888, melancholics accounted for 33 per cent of the year's total admissions, with a recovery rate of 27 per cent.

The general unreliability of accompanying evidence was problematic when assigning the patients' causes of insanity and understanding the true nature of the illness. In 1876 Brushfield complained bitterly that the involvement of the Poor Law relieving officer in the clerical process had led to 'defective and even perverted histories of the cases' being given to the medical officers so that there was no idea of the cause of insanity for two-thirds of Brookwood patients.[25] This was similar to Exminster, where a sampling of the 1880–2 admissions records shows that in almost two-thirds of cases, the cause of insanity was either not known or not provided.[26] Melling has partially attributed this to certifying doctors being either unable or unwilling to identify a specific cause of their patients' insanity.

As part of the Brookwood management's efforts to maintain more informative patient records as required by the Commissioners in Lunacy, the asylum began to try to systematically record and tabulate causes of insanity, broadly dividing them into moral and physical types, so that, by 1890, only a quarter of Brookwood patients had no cause cited for their condition.

The primary 'moral' causes for all Brookwood patients, whether 'predisposing or exciting' were similar to those recorded at Holloway. 'Mental worry of various kinds' was the primary cause, closely followed by 'domestic trouble' (including bereavement of family or friends), and 'adverse circumstances', such as business worries and pecuniary problems. Religious excitement and 'love affairs, including seduction' were also frequently cited in the records, but usually as the 'exciting' precipitator of the patient's current bout of insanity.

Intemperance, bodily disease, previous attacks and hereditary insanity featured amongst the physical causes.[27] Intemperance as a primary cause was common to both men and women, but in 1895 more cases than usual were ascribed to alcoholic dependence: 50 cases, or 18 per cent of admissions. Some patients took to alcohol as a result of financial or domestic difficulties, such as unemployment or desertion by a husband. Others had sustained and long-term excessive drinking habits, such as Thomas H., who arrived at Brookwood in April 1878. Something of a local celebrity, the former Surrey cricketer-turned-publican was reported to have 'been a hard drinker for years and has frequently suffered from Delirium Tremens'. Weak and delusional, he died within five months of his admission.[28]

The link with hereditary causes was acknowledged infrequently before the late 1880s. Reporting on the 286 patients admitted to Brookwood in 1895, however, the superintendent remarked that, in his opinion, 'hereditary taint' existed in nearly a third, and throughout the 1890s, this remained a fairly consistent diagnosis. He had traced the lineage where possible, in both male and female cases, and ascertained that insanity was equally likely to be transferred directly from mothers or fathers. At a time when the mechanisms of inheritance were not fully understood, he also claimed that it had been transferred from brothers and sisters in twenty new cases admitted in 1895.[29]

At Holloway Sanatorium, although the assigned causes were broadly similar, abject poverty featured less, but reduced circumstances or work troubles were not uncommon. The origins or causes of the patients' insanity were discussed frequently in the superintendent's annual reports. Worry and anxiety over business, overwork and domestic troubles were all seen as triggers for insanity, and accounted for nearly one-third of admissions in most years. In 1890, Rees Philipps remarked that 'In a third of the cases also some hereditary taint of insanity was ascertained, and in a large number of cases, heredity and worry were associated as predisposing and exciting causes respectively'. One case believed to be of hereditary origin was Ellen B., who was admitted to Holloway at the age of nineteen, diagnosed as an 'adolescent melancholic'. She was brought from her home in Kew by her father, who himself had suffered from an attack of mania three years previously. The cause of Ellen's insanity was seen as being solely hereditary; her father's illness was cited as evidence, and it was also alleged that Ellen's maternal grandmother had suffered from melancholia.[30] Hereditary causes continued to be associated with approximately a third of the Holloway admissions during the years under study (until 1905).

Alcoholic intemperance was attributed to a smaller number of cases at Holloway than at Brookwood; for example, in 1890, it was cited as a cause in only 8 per cent of cases.[31] The superintendent consistently reinforced his belief that 'worry' was 'the most potent cause of insanity' amongst his patients. Contrary to Dr Clouston's observations of his patients at Morningside Asylum in Edinburgh (which led him to believe that alcohol was the chief case of insanity), Rees Philipps believed that intemperance was more likely to be a product of insanity as opposed to a cause.[32]

Principles and Proponents of Moral Treatment

Treatment in the nineteenth century was based on principles of protective custody. It began with the separation of the patient from society, either voluntary or enforced, and placement within designated facilities. Within specialized accommodation – the asylum – the intention was to bring about a cure, a fundamental principle that stemmed from practices at Bethlem and other charitable and subscription asylums.[33] Patients' removal from their current environment was viewed by the medical profession as critical, since it was believed that families and friends, no matter how well intentioned, could have a detrimental influence on the patient's mental condition. Ideally, the patient was removed as soon as possible for treatment so as to facilitate an early, and potentially full, recovery. Regulated, well-managed and secure accommodation endorsed the medical theory of separation, and justified the existence of the asylum as the appropriate environment for custodial treatment.

Once in the asylum, patients were subjected to constant scrutiny and a structured therapeutic routine that included work, amusements and possibly chemical intervention, although the latter was not a core constituent of moral therapy. Broadly, moral treatment embraced a collection of non-medical treatments (unless deemed as unavoidable), rather than one specific technique, and also sought to involve patients in their own recovery process. This was the basis of most treatment of the insane from the early to mid-nineteenth century, by which time mechanical restraint, which had been subject to much criticism, was formally abolished in many public and private institutions. The treatment of the nineteenth-century lunatic was widely acknowledged to be all-encompassing:

> Under this head should be included all that relates to the management of the lunatic, from the moment that it is determined that he shall be removed to an asylum until his career as a patient ends, by discharge on recovery, removal, or death.[34]

Whilst it had not originated at the York Retreat, which opened in 1796, moral treatment had become closely associated with this particular institution, as part of a more compassionate approach to the treatment of lunatics that was adopted and actively promoted by the Tuke family. The primary focus was on the rational and the emotional causes of insanity rather than any organic origins. Self-discipline, and thus mastery over one's illness, was fundamental.[35] A more formalized adoption of the principles of moral treatments was later promoted by John Conolly at Hanwell, Robert Gardner Hill at Lincoln, and John Bucknill at Exeter.[36] The environment was extremely important, and although it had to be secure, it also aimed to be comfortable and civilized, with attractive grounds to lift the spirits and distract patients from any melancholic thoughts or associations. Taking the environment alone, Holloway's opulence was without question, but even Brookwood, a sprawling and crowded county asylum, managed to achieve an air of domesticity with its pleasant, well-planned grounds and attention to interior details. Despite initial difficulties in achieving this, by 1877 commentators observed that 'The visitor to Brookwood will be strongly impressed by its simple homely characteristics'.[37]

Christian values were an important component of moral therapy, not least because they had the potential to instil a fear of wrongdoing, and so arguably assisted patients in exercising self-restraint. The Commissioners in Lunacy insisted a chapel was provided by all asylums, which from 1887 had to be detached from the main building, and able to hold at least three-quarters of the patients.[38] It was thought that the chaplain and his services could benefit the diseased mind, provided that both the chapel and the sermons were adapted appropriately for their specialized congregation. This included a veto on any mention of death. The commissioners' advice was that cheerfulness was essential:

> The airs of the pulpit are wholly out of place in an asylum; its graces should be cultivated, because none are too poor to be pleased. Sometimes one hears a sermon from an asylum pulpit so prosy, so ill-judged, and above all so monotonous, that it must take a week of pleasant intercourse with patients to wipe it out of memory.[39]

The chaplain's role, whilst non-medical, was therefore of considerable importance. This was reflected in his position within the asylum staff hierarchy and the fact that his remuneration was second only to that of the medical superintendent at both asylums.

As an all-encompassing benign and humane approach, moral treatment was principally aimed at the 'moral', or psychological and emotional faculties of the patients. Self-regulation, as opposed to coercive discipline, was promoted. It has been suggested that, although hereditary insanity and the association with incurability had been identified by earlier alienists, an emphasis on moral causes remained. This essentially optimistic approach was later eroded by an increased interest in eugenics amongst the medical community and others. The tendency to adopt a eugenic and hereditary perspective to insanity implied a poor prognosis.[40] This more pessimistic approach towards the care and custody of the insane gathered momentum as the century progressed.

General Therapeutics

'Medical' treatment was not confined to the administration of medicines and pills; Dr Brushfield, and medical observers such as Mortimer Granville, believed that the medical treatment for the insane could not exist in isolation, but must encompass every aspect of their daily care and management under the superintendent and his staff. Brushfield was particularly vigilant in this respect: 'The policy has been to place the inmates of Brookwood asylum as nearly as may be amidst the surroundings of sane life, and then to treat them as children under a perpetual personal guardianship'.[41] A safe and comfortable environment was complemented by a manageable degree of stimulation and the grounds were essential for regular exercise for those who were able. Asylum grounds (whether pauper or private) were primarily based on the country house model, but modified to address the needs of an extensive building usually located in a rural setting. This needed to be decorative to provide a visual distraction, but it had to offer the potential for agricultural self-sufficiency.[42]

Moral therapeutic treatment at Brookwood was occasionally compromised by the building work undertaken to provide more patient accommodation, yet Brushfield continually strove to elevate Brookwood's status beyond that of a mere large custodial institution. He used the expansion programmes as opportunities to secure additional features to improve the therapeutic facilities for his patients. His great success was to gain agreement for the construction of a large, purpose-built recreational hall that had been omitted from the original design. This was operational from 1874 and made possible a much improved entertainments programme for the patients. As noted, Holloway also was obliged to expand and provide more accommodation for both patients and staff alike.[43] Naturally, this building work was disruptive to the sanatorium's daily regime, and, occasionally, having workmen on the premises proved to be extremely dangerous. Doors and windows were left unsecured, equipment was left unattended, and the workmen fraternized with the patients. Tragically, a rope carelessly left by workmen in the Great Hall enabled one elderly melancholic female patient to hang herself in 1887.[44]

The mutual relationship between the body and the mind, the need to protect yet cure, the interconnectedness of the lives of staff and patients, and the relationship of both within the therapeutic environment, caused some confusion in asylums. For example, seclusion was essentially a method of physical restraint, although the asylums allegedly operated within policies of non-restraint, indicating that – to some extent – this term was a misnomer. As contemporaries recognized, practically or legally, the procedure would otherwise have been more accurately described as retirement, implying patient consent and therefore negating any need for restraint.[45] Although he acknowledged that seclusion was occasionally unavoidable at Brookwood, Brushfield advocated that outdoor occupation was much the best approach for the most difficult patients.[46] The extensive grounds offered plenty of opportunities for agricultural pursuits that were particularly suited to the men. The asylum became self-sufficient and profitable from selling its excess produce, as well as taking in laundry from other nearby institutions. By 1875, large areas of Brookwood's land had been successfully cultivated and regularly maintained by the patients. There were potato and vegetable fields, kitchen and flower gardens, strawberry beds and orchards. Patients also worked on the farm or in one of the workshops, assisting the joiner, the upholsterer, the baker or the bricklayer.

As seen earlier, 'work as therapy' was segregated by gender, as asylums were operated primarily on a domestic model. Thus, female patients were primarily employed in the kitchen, the laundry and the sewing room, where they made and repaired patients' clothing, stockings and bed linen. They also worked in the wards (as did a few men). Every effort was made to ensure that the majority of patients were kept gainfully employed in and around the asylum in one capacity or another. This policy was largely successful; in 1870 for example, only one-eighth of all patients was unfit for physical work.[47] Annual reports continually showed that at least two-thirds of the patients worked, and that they made a positive contribution to agriculture and gardening, as well as maintaining the internal and external decoration of the asylum. Work was also a means of measuring the patients' recovery, in that those who worked harder were judged to be recovering more quickly than 'indolent' patients, who were observed to be not making so much progress.[48]

At Holloway, patients were also encouraged to work, although not to the same extent as at Brookwood. There was general agreement that some forms of labour were inappropriate for particular patients, given their class and status. However, idleness was seen as dangerous and the therapeutic value of physical work recognized, so a few workshops were established to encourage patient participation. Uptake of work was generally slow; in 1888 the Commissioners in Lunacy reported that only thirty-six male patients were working, mostly in the kitchen garden and on the farmland.[49] Outdoor employment schemes for the men were set up early on, but similar schemes for the women were less successful; although many of them were capable, there was reluctance to take part. By 1890, this situation had begun to change, forty-three men were working outside and '30 others are induced to occupy themselves in useful ways'.[50] Encouragingly, forty-three female patients were employed in general housework duties around the sanatorium. A further sixty-six women were sufficiently trusted to be allowed to take up needlework and knitting. This meant that over half the resident females were being kept regularly occupied, and this remained consistent for the next ten years. Many patients' activities at Holloway were not formally regulated, unlike at Brookwood where working parties were clocked in and out, and details of morning and afternoon activities scheduled and routinely recorded. The laundry had always been regarded as a useful place to employ women in asylums and prisons, but, at the sanatorium, it was regarded as an unsuitable environment for patients, particularly women, until after 1896, when a major refurbishment increased the safety levels. Then it offered valuable therapeutic benefits to all classes of patients, even the voluntary boarders.

Patients were exercised daily in the grounds of both institutions, although fewer women took part and all difficult or feeble patients were restricted to short periods in the airing courts. The occasional building work constrained exercise and sporting activities, which made life more difficult for medical staff; exercise was not only therapeutic but it also tired the patients and made them more malleable. At Holloway, some patients were allowed the privilege of walking unattended inside (or even beyond) the sanatorium grounds and they occasionally made short excursions to local shops and facilities. If they were physically feeble, there was the option of carriage rides around the local countryside, either using their own transport or that provided by the sanatorium. Clearly, this was not a facility that was available to Brookwood's patients.

Brookwood's moral treatment did have its lighter side, however; regular and wide-ranging entertainments were held at the asylum. These were (certainly initially) rather more 'home-grown' and of a less sophisticated character than those at Holloway. This was especially so before the recreation hall was built, when only four out of a whole programme of events were provided by paid entertainers.[51] The new hall allowed at least one or two amusements every week, such as 'readings, concerts, Christy minstrels, the marionettes, conjuring entertainments, dissolving views, dialogues, extravaganzas, plays and pantomimes'.[52] Staff, together with patients, often designed and participated in concerts, recitals or plays, including Brushfield: 'He was not only a successful director of the institution, but play writer, composer, stage manager, and actor of no mean capacity'.[53] Events were well attended by both staff and patients and they also served as an excellent public relations exercise, as audiences regularly included the county's gentry, doctors, clergy and military officers.

Brushfield's achievements within a public asylum were recognized as innovative and creative: 'His kind and thoughtful solicitude for the welfare of his unfortunate patients caused him to promote schemes for their entertainment which have been adopted in every asylum since that time'.[54] His recreational innovations had begun while he was at Chester, and contemporaries observed that they were 'part of a system, his system at least of the treatment of the insane with a view to their recovery or improvement'.[55] The annual fancy-dress balls were sufficiently novel to warrant press attention and were praised as being indicative of Brushfield's 'high reputation in the practice of psychological medical treatment'.[56] In 1881, the *Illustrated London News* reported that 400 costumed patients and staff had attended the fancy-dress ball for which the sixteen-piece Asylum Band played, and that the recreation hall was 'beautifully decorated with exotic plants, flags, wreaths, statuettes, mirrors, and Chinese lanterns'. Later, the Eighteenth Royal Irish Regiment played as a further 200 visitors arrived, and after midnight refreshments, the patients were removed, leaving the local dignitaries to frolic for several more hours.[57]

As part of Holloway's therapeutic regime, patients were encouraged to follow the middle-class lifestyle that they supposedly enjoyed prior to admission. George Martin Holloway wrote that it had been the intention of his illustrious relative to provide the sanatorium patients with 'all the elegancies of a refined House'.[58] In some instances, asylum life provided patients with a better standard of living than they were used to 'outside'. The sanatorium's design and facilities were part of this approach to caring for the middle-class insane and they were constantly reviewed to ensure the best was being provided; one example was the introduction of a table d'hôte dinner from 1889 for those well enough to attend, which was held at 6.30 pm with tea and music. Every suitable recreational facility imaginable was made available to the patients. There were tennis courts (flooded in winter for skating), a billiards room, cricket and football pitches, a gymnasium and a swimming pool in the summer months. Despite the introduction of the gymnasium and the pool facilities for the patients, there is no evidence that they were part of a regulated therapeutic regime.[59] The medical superintendent favoured hydrotherapy for treating mania and regretted that it could not be used, as technically it was considered a form of mechanical restraint.[60]

Holloway had an annual athletic sports day that included the usual competitions, together with light-hearted events such as an egg and spoon race. The sanatorium's sports teams competed with other hospitals and institutions throughout the year. The superintendent's annual reports recorded all the activities; for example in 1895, there were picnics, dances, smoking concerts, theatricals and lectures as well as the sporting competitions.[61] Rees Philipps stated that all the events and facilities were available to voluntary and certified patients alike, regardless of their financial or charitable status. Maniacal patients were, however, prohibited. The sanatorium's management particularly valued the musical and sporting skills of their doctors, attendants and companions, as the teams, choirs and bands frequently constituted both patients and staff, and made local public appearances which strengthened their relationship with the surrounding community.

Rees Philipps pointed out that sufficient horses and carriages were essential given the sanatorium's rural location. They were used for general excursions as well as providing carriage rides for infirm patients who would otherwise remain indoors.[62] For the more sedentary, there was the library, art classes, photography and needlework, the results of which were proudly displayed in exhibitions such as the one held in December 1899. Encouraged by the medical staff, the patients issued the first edition of their own magazine, *St Ann's*, in 1894, which contained poems, articles and anecdotes that jostled with reports of annual tennis tournaments and cricket and football matches.[63] The production of this magazine was facilitated by a new printing press in 1899, which allowed the sanatorium to print all their theatre, dance and concert programmes, 'monthly calendars' and any other items they needed.[64] In 1896, *St Ann's* reported on the annual athletics sports day, noting that spectators included 'numerous friends from the outside', thus indicating the centrality and status of the sanatorium within the local community, with events such as these being open to the general public.[65]

Some patients were trusted to organize their own independent social life, often assisted by their personal servants so that they enjoyed a certain amount of freedom. The superintendent described the asylum's approach to its middle-class inmates: 'the utmost liberty, consistent with safety, is permitted'.[66] Wealthier patients were allowed shopping excursions to London and to attend events such the Henley Regatta and horse racing at Ascot and Epsom. There were regular river trips to local beauty spots such as Windsor, Marlow or Taplow Woods. Holloway patients and boarders also benefited from seaside air when they were sent to the sanatorium's secondary branch for anything up to two months at a time. Initially this was rented accommodation in Torquay and Ramsgate, but later a small villa was purchased at Hove, and was efficiently run by Mrs Rees Philipps.[67] The voluntary patients occasionally abused the management's trust, and in so doing, arguably sabotaged their own chances of recovery. One female patient was admitted in November 1891 during which time she continued with her 'self-destructive' daily habit of a bottle of chlorodyne and several cigars. During her five-week stay, she refused to be examined and defied any restrictions so that she could still make regular visits to the nearby shops to collect her supplies.[68]

The philosophy of resocialization as part of a range of appropriate therapeutics for middle-class patients prompted the employment of the lady and gentlemen companions. It also led to the decision that, unless medically disadvantageous, patients' relatives could stay at the sanatorium if they wished. Some patients benefited from this and the practice had the additional advantages of demonstrating the humane treatment regime while providing welcome additional income. It appears to have been a relatively popular scheme, with as many as forty-five residential visitors recorded in 1887.[69]

Physical Treatments

The extent and impact of the use of specific treatments is difficult to assess, given the nature of asylum sources. In particular, the patient's view of their own treatment is rarely accessible, as most of the evidence is from official sources and the perspective of senior medical staff. Annual reports recorded numbers of cured patients, as these were of particular interest as a measure of success, often to explicitly compare one institution to another. Individual treatments were sometimes recorded in the patient's case book but recordkeeping was inconsistent and unreliable. Case books were regularly updated in the early stages of a patient's stay but, as has been pointed out, if they became long-term or chronic inmates, entries were often perfunctory with just enough detail to ensure legality and recertification.[70]

In accordance with therapeutic practice in other asylums, both Brookwood and Holloway encouraged their patients to achieve self-control. At the most basic level, this could mean punishment for transgression and reward for compliance. Unacceptable or difficult behaviour could mean seclusion from the other inmates, and being barred from participation in the institution's daily life. Catherine H. was admitted to Brookwood in June 1871 suffering from mania. She was a difficult patient whose suicidal and violent behaviour was treated with hemp and digitalis, but this was largely ineffective. She was repeatedly segregated but never left entirely alone as she was constantly accompanied by a delegated nurse. Occasionally, she recovered sufficiently and behaved well enough to be allowed to rejoin the other patients at work or in recreation. However, she usually reverted to violence within a short space of time and attacked patients and staff. She frequently damaged asylum property and, after breaking the windows for a second time, the staff cut off her hair as a punishment.[71] This was not an isolated type of reprimand, although occasionally such action was taken primarily for medical purposes, such as in the case of Catherine M., admitted in 1876. Although she was a difficult patient and had received chemical therapy, she had her hair cut off to ease the effects of a rash.[72]

Seclusion was used to contain violent outbursts and also to protect staff and other patients. Patients were secluded until they had mastered their behaviour. It was essential that standards of patient discipline were maintained, as an unruly patient unsettled other patients, caused additional work for the staff and was a potential danger to themselves or others. Brushfield believed that seclusion was best defined as follows:

> Whenever a patient is placed during the day in any room or locality, *alone and with locked doors*, the case may be viewed and recorded as one of seclusion, irrespectively altogether of the question whether seclusion was adopted for purposes of medical treatment or for purposes of discipline.[73]

He attributed the high incidence of seclusion during Brookwood's first year to the fact that the asylum was new and had problems recruiting constant staff. Of the forty-nine cases of seclusion recorded that year, thirty-six were women suffering from puerperal mania. Brushfield described one patient (who prior to admission had been treated with opium) as the worst case he had ever seen during his medical career.[74] However, patients continued to be secluded for short periods following 'ordinary' quarrelling, or for minor insubordination. Brushfield openly regretted that annoying an attendant often led to a patient being locked away as this gave the impression of seclusion as punishment and not medical treatment. This 'ordinary seclusion' he regarded as dubious moral treatment since it was 'little better than neglect by leaving the patient to his own resources'.[75]

In order to remove a patient suffering with an episode of mental excitement it was necessary to use a degree of physical coercion. Given the stated aim of using as little restraint as possible, it might be assumed that this was minimal. The patient would be forcibly removed from his or her current environment and usually placed alone in a bedroom or a padded room. Brookwood had no padded rooms fitted until 1885, and Holloway had one padded room for female patients and installed another in the male side of the Retreat (the unit for excitable patients) in 1889.[76] When the temporary removal of a patient was perceived as unavoidable, Brushfield ordered his staff to follow an unusual and particular strategy whereby the patient was placed in a room with one to three attendants rather than be locked up alone. Gradually, the attendants would leave, until only one remained. This last member of staff would withdraw, leaving the door ajar. If the patient fell asleep, the door was closed, but left unlocked. Brushfield believed that his modified practice was infinitely preferable to sole exclusion, as it 'secures safety to the patient and takes away all excuse for negligence on the part of the attendant'.[77]

The Holloway records show that seclusion was used often, but the register of incidents has not survived, so its nature cannot be accurately determined. The Commissioners in Lunacy, visiting the sanatorium in December 1888, noted that no one was in seclusion, and that just one man and woman had been restrained, and 'they were only gloved'.[78] By October 1890, however, eleven men had been secluded on 49 occasions for a total of 299 hours, and four women on 31 occasions for 228 hours. In addition, other forms of what can only be termed as 'restraint' were also practised; three patients had been 'wet-packed' for a total of 36 hours, two restrained by 'sleeve jacket' for a total of 30 hours, and a further seven patients subjected to 'locked gloves' for 169 hours in all.[79] Suicidal and self-harming patients were often restrained by a straitjacket. Evelyn Mary S., aged forty-three, arrived at the sanatorium in April 1903 and after several vicious attempts at self-harm (including trying to gouge out her eyes), was reported to have spent a total of 55¾ hours in a long-sleeved jacket during May that year; this was an average of nearly two hours each day.[80]

The failure of one restraint method known as 'dry-pack' ultimately led to the death of a 24-year-old patient in 1894. Thomas W., an engineer, was transferred to Holloway on 17 July from Hoxton House. Initially described as suffering from melancholia, his condition deteriorated and by 26 July he was suffering from 'maniacal excitement with violence'. To manage this, he was restrained in a dry-pack on several occasions, up to nine hours at any one time. During the week leading up to his death on the 30 September, he had been restrained for as much as eighteen hours a day. The dry-pack was described as follows:

> The apparatus consists of a blanket and five broad leather straps, connected at intervals by loops with two strips of webbing about six feet in length. The patient is laid upon the blanket, which is drawn over him and folded so as to envelop him tightly from head to foot. He is then laid upon one of the strips of webbing, and the other is brought down the centre of the front of his body, and the straps are drawn suffi-

ciently tight to restrain the movements of all his limbs and keep his arms close to his sides. The upper part of the blanket is then sewn back to prevent interference with respiration by the nose and mouth, and the two lower ends of the webbing are tied between the feet. It all together depends on the degree in which the straps are tightened whether or not there is interference with the necessary movements of the chest for respiratory purposes, and with the circulation.[81]

Holloway Sanatorium was strongly criticized by the Commissioners in Lunacy for the way it mismanaged this case. It also came under attack from the popular press, partially fuelled by the accusations of the young man's father that the sanatorium had also abused its charitable status.[82] He claimed that the institution had attempted to extort additional fees from Thomas's family for his care, and that when these were not forthcoming, Rees Philipps had placed his son in this fatal restraint.[83] The Commissioners in Lunacy concentrated on the practical mismanagement of the case, highlighting the too-tight straps that prevented the patient from breathing properly, the fact that he was left unattended for lengthy periods, and the inadequate supervision. As a result of the inquest, the contraption was outlawed in all asylums, and a modified version (without the straps) was introduced. Despite the two inquests and the negative publicity, there is no evidence that families removed their relatives as a result of the fatality, nor was there any reduction in the numbers of admissions.[84]

Holloway continually tried to provide a curative regime suitable for its middle-class clientele, and to offer better and more up-to-date facilities than its competitors. Consideration was given habitually to new and innovative treatments that were rarely, if ever, used at Brookwood, or were not introduced until a later date. For example, electric therapy was in use at the sanatorium from *c.* 1886, although details are scant. Electrotherapy does not appear to have been in common use in many public asylums at this time, but it gradually increased in popularity before the First World War. Some doctors preferred faradic, or interrupted current, and others galvanic, or continued current. Patients could be immersed in galvanic baths or wear belts, and electricity was applied to virtually any part of the body.[85] At Holloway, it appears to have been used irregularly and usually after other methods of physical and chemical treatment had been tried with no discernible success. Typical were cases of severe melancholia that were accompanied by suicidal tendencies.[86] The first reference traced at Brookwood occurred in 1893, when galvanization, in conjunction with morphine and quinine, was applied to a 33-year-old patient, Agnes C., who had been diagnosed with uterine-induced mania.[87] Other less aggressive physical treatments employed for Holloway patients included massage, gymnastic classes and a Turkish bath for male patients.[88] A swimming pool was built and made available for the patients' supervised use from 1896.

Chemical and Medical Treatments

Although the York Retreat, the most influential of voluntary asylums, was strongly associated with moral treatment, it also carried out a limited range of medical interventions. By the mid-nineteenth century, the principles of non-restraint had been ostensibly adopted by most institutions (although not always reflected in reality), so that asylum superintendents were obliged to consider other methods of management and treatment, particularly for dealing with excitable or violent patients. Despite having established comprehensive work and entertainment schedules for the patients, there were evidently occasions when these proved ineffective to distract or cure. At Brookwood, in particular, financial constraints limited available medication, and many patients were not treated chemically unless the severity of their symptoms and subsequent manageability made it unavoidable. The extent of chemical intervention is difficult to ascertain; but, at both institutions, medical staff utilized a limited pharmacopoeia for certain patients, particularly (although not exclusively) those who exhibited violent or suicidal tendencies. These patients, who were primarily a danger to themselves, could cause other patients to mimic their behaviour.

Eating disorders, frequently associated with suicidal tendency and melancholia, are recorded more frequently in the Holloway case books than at Brookwood. Such behaviour may have been more apparent at Holloway due to the higher staff-to-patient ratios and the use of the 'companions' who mixed so closely with the patients. Many Brookwood patients had previously suffered financial deprivation and, once in the asylum, benefited from a relatively good diet which was central to the therapeutic regime. Dietary 'extras' were provided for weak or ailing patients at both institutions, and they were regularly weighed as part of the ongoing assessment of their mental and physical health.

Some patients harboured delusions about food (that it was poisoned, for example) or refused food as part of their suicidal inclination, meaning they had to be occasionally fed by the attendants. Not wishing to eat, or even drink, may have been the result of some individualized protest, but such behaviour might not have constituted a full-blown eating disorder.[89] At Holloway, Anne, a 33-year-old spinster, was regularly admitted suffering from violent mania. She had attempted to escape on two occasions, and regularly refused food, so that the attendants had no option other than to tube-feed her three times daily. Apparently violent, she 'does not make the slightest resistance to the operation, walks quietly in, sits down to have it performed, opens her mouth voluntarily so that the gag is almost unnecessary'.[90] It was more usual for patients to resist, as did one diminutive young woman who put up such a struggle that it required several attendants to hold her down and introduce the feeding tube.[91] For some late nineteenth-century clinicians, the association of food-denial with melancholia and suicidal propensity meant that prompt intervention was seen as crucial. It has also been suggested that appetite disorders were reputed to have associations with masturbation and sexuality, although there is not a reference to this at Brookwood and Holloway.[92]

Both asylums applied 'blisters' to patients, often, although not exclusively, on male patients in cases where masturbation had been observed. They could be applied to the genitals or to the back of the neck. This was a long-established practice in asylums and was intended to produce a counter-irritant that diverted the mind.[93] At Ticehurst, counter-irritations were prescribed for cases of acute mania and excessive masturbation.[94] For 26-year-old Henry H., admitted to Brookwood in 1871 with mania, his constant masturbation meant that this device was applied to his prepuce many times, but neither this, nor digitalis, deterred him from his habit, nor from his many attempts to escape.[95]

Large numbers of allegedly suicidal patients were admitted to both asylums.[96] At Brookwood, many patients originating from the urban workhouses were described as 'suicidal', and it is highly possible that this terminology was used to facilitate the transfer of difficult inmates to the county asylum for the convenience of workhouse masters. Often these cases arrived bound in straight-jackets, or strong dresses, but exhibited no self-destructive tendencies once under treatment in the asylum. Dr Brushfield believed that all melancholics were at risk, women especially, but his primary policy of intense surveillance seems to have been successful, with only three recorded suicides during this period.[97] Surveillance was also the main preventative at Holloway but it was employed with reluctance on the part of the superintendent, who believed that constant observation was just as likely to irritate patients, and could actually hinder their recovery. Suicidal 'accidents' he felt were inevitable; in fact, if there were none, this indicated that the supervision was too strict.[98] But these patients were not left totally untreated, and the Holloway case books indicate that those who exhibited violent or suicidal tendencies received more physical and chemical interventions. These included combinations of digitalis, bromide, hypodermic morphia, purgatives and electricity.

At Brookwood, the first two medical superintendents preferred to prescribe moral order, fresh air and employment but there was still a place for some limited chemical intervention. The evidence indicates that the routine administration of drugs was restricted, partially due to costs, but also because so many cases were seen as incurable and therefore unlikely to warrant the investment.[99] However, it is difficult to assess the scope of chemical intervention, not least because of poor recording methods that came under fire from the Commissioners in Lunacy in 1868.

Given Brookwood's size and the superintendent's workload, it is not surprising to uncover incidences where medication was used to induce compliance and order, especially where patients had a history of violent and disruptive behaviour. Mortimer Granville had suggested that drugs were widely employed in asylums under the guise of scientific and humane practice in the age of non-restraint.[100] Chloral, opium, hyoscyamus or digitalis were sometimes used at Brookwood during patients' periods of mental excitement so as to conserve the patient's strength, particularly if they were distressed and agitated upon arrival, or if persistently violent or actively suicidal.[101] The reality of institutional treatment was, Granville declared, that 'the pretence of curative treatment was a sophistry' and the use of these drugs and other sedatives was 'a most mischievous form of restraint' used to obtain quiet and orderly wards.[102] However, there is no evidence that Brushfield or his successor adopted such a policy; contemporary witnesses suggest the opposite, and in his extensive survey of asylum care, Granville firmly declared that Brushfield did not believe in the use of drugs 'to produce quiet'.[103] Brushfield may have been unusual in this regard. Whilst medication was usually used for the more refractory inmates, it was suspended if favourable results were not seen quickly. Elizabeth K. was first admitted in 1867 aged ten, and during this and her many subsequent readmissions, she was subjected to a wide-ranging (and seemingly random), array of treatments that included morphine, potassium bromide, cold water baths and periods of solitary confinement. She had also been given dietary supplements (eggs and brandy) but this was stopped, as it 'made her stronger to do evil'. Her medication was also halted when it was seen that her behaviour remained unchanged.[104]

Rather surprisingly for a public asylum, the Brookwood doctors performed surgery on a female patient after treatment with potassium bromide had failed to relieve her symptoms.[105] Augusta S., a 39-year-old married woman from Dorking, was admitted in October 1890 suffering from mania with suspected symptoms of GPI, allegedly caused by drink. Her husband reported that, previously, she had sustained a blow to the top of her head as she climbed out of the cellar, and this was noted as a predisposing cause of insanity. When she arrived at Brookwood, she was delusional, generally incoherent and expressed 'exalted' ideas, symptoms which worsened by February 1891. Around this date, Augusta's husband gave his consent for a surgical procedure to be carried out on his wife and later that month, Dr Gayton, assisted by Dr Barton, performed 'the operation of trepanning'.[106] This was pronounced a success by the doctors and Augusta was discharged as recovered in June 1891.[107]

At Holloway Sanatorium, hypnotics, sedatives and laxatives were more routinely dispensed to patients; some details of these have survived.[108] Many were given to relieve bodily ailments, or to treat various general disorders, such as diarrhoea, gout, eye infections or coughs and colds.[109] Epsom salts and Vaseline were also dispensed. Tonics, either in liquid or tablet form, were given to patients to increase their appetite, or for general improvement of bodily conditions that were believed to act adversely on the mind, such as constipation or irregular periods.

While some constituents and drugs are now known to be ineffective or even dangerous, they were administered at the time in accordance with current medical practice, and in the belief that every weapon should be used in the battle against insanity. A few remedies have survived and proved their therapeutic value, albeit in a different capacity. The quantities of active ingredients used are unclear, as often concoctions used volumes of tinctures or aqueous solutions so that the concentrations of the actual drug cannot be ascertained. It is possible that doses of hazardous substances, such as arsenic or strychnine, were relatively small, in spite of them being the main components of some tonics. For example, arsenic mixed with potassium and ammonium bromide produced a mild, but potentially dangerous, sedative frequently administered at Holloway. One favourite appetite stimulant contained gentian (traditionally known for this property) along with sodium bicarbonate, but it also contained arsenic and strychnine.[110] The dispensary records do not clarify what symptoms or diagnosis led to medicines being dispensed, although occasionally some case notes for suicidal and violent patients have recorded this information.

Opiates such as morphia and opium were commonly deployed both inside and outside the asylum in the nineteenth century. Many patent medicines contained opium and its medical use had been important for some time. It was the stuff of 'infant doping' in preparations such as Godfrey's Cordial, and was also used recreationally, and as an everyday remedy for common ailments.[111] It soon evolved into an asylum staple, and, as Digby has pointed out, it was referred to in contemporary text books as 'the sheet anchor of the alienist physician'.[112]

In the asylum, opium could be mixed in peppermint water; morphine with chloroform (chlorodyne) was also regularly used. A tablespoon of cocaine (in water) was administered three times daily to one patient, and it was also a prime constituent in an often-dispensed mixture alongside capsicum (an extract of cayenne pepper) and strychnine. Inducement of sleep was vital for patient strength and recovery, and was beneficial to the smooth running of any asylum regime. Sulphonal (a trade name for sulphonmethane) was a hypnotic that was frequently prescribed and seen in many case books, as was paraldehyde, also used for its hypnotic and sedative properties. Yet another sedative mixture was potassium bromide together with hyoscine.[113] These medications would have arguably helped relieve anxiety or calmed patients and perhaps helped them sleep.[114]

Outcomes

Brookwood's management repeatedly blamed the asylum's low recovery rates on the receipt of so many workhouse inmates in poor physical and mental condition. Although this may have been exaggerated, it reflects the evidence from other county asylum superintendents that new patients often arrived weakened by poverty, malnutrition and disease, reducing their ability to improve. For example, the Devon County Asylum reported that patients admitted from the nearby Plympton workhouse were substantially less likely to recover than those sent from home.[115]

Table 5.1: Summary of total admissions to Brookwood, 1867–85.

Percentage of cases	Males	Females	Both sexes
Recovered	28.5	33.0	30.08
Relieved	4.5	4.2	4.3
Died	32.6	23.7	28.0
Remaining	15.5	20.7	18.3
Total	**100.0**	**100.0**	**100.0**

Source: Reproduced from the Nineteenth Annual Report of the Committee of Visitors to the Surrey County Lunatic Asylum at Brookwood for 1885.[116]

Brookwood's management calculated that, from 1867 to 1885, the average recovery rate for all patients stood at just over 30 per cent with slightly better outcomes for the women who either were discharged quickly or remained in the asylum for many years (Table 5.1).[117] Men were more susceptible to death in in custody, with just over 32 per cent during these years as opposed to nearly 24 per cent of women. This endorses the findings of Wright on Buckinghamshire County Asylum.[118] Ray's earlier research has also highlighted that the fast turnover of county asylum patients was overlooked by historians who he believed were preoccupied with institutionalization and the accumulation of incurable cases.[119]

Brushfield believed that the admission of general paralytics adversely affected Brookwood's recovery rates, as the condition had a poor prognosis. GPI produced severe symptoms which required more intensive nursing and so was a considerable drain on medical resources. There was confusion regarding the causes of GPI; syphilis had been suggested as early as 1857 but this was not generally accepted at this time. Rather, the condition was believed to result from several interlinked causes that derived from an urban environment and its associated iniquities, such as excessive alcohol consumption and sexual promiscuity.[120] There was more general agreement regarding the physical symptoms which included inarticulate speech, tremulous lips and tongue, progressive muscular paralysis and inevitable fatality. Classically, patients exhibited delusions of grandeur accompanied by either mania or dementia, but medical confusion remained and as Davis has pointed out, an informed diagnosis could not truly be given until the final stages of the disease and death confirmed the diagnosis.[121]

It has been estimated that, in the nineteenth century, up to 20 per cent of British men admitted to English asylums were diagnosed as suffering from GPI. These cases invariably died shortly after admission (other than in a few cases of misdiagnosis where the patient was miraculously cured).[122] The *Lancet* observed that, between June 1867 and December 1874, this disease accounted for 31.35 per cent of Brookwood's total mortality, or 140 out of 451 deaths in all. GPI was held to be the primary cause of death for just under half of all male deaths but for only 1 per cent of female mortality.[123] One case in every 8.5 inmates was a sufferer, which compared unfavourably with the larger first county asylum at Wandsworth, where it was one in 22.4.[124] When only five known GPI patients were admitted to Brookwood in 1890, the medical superintendent James Barton attributed this to the fact that they had only received new cases from rural Surrey that year, so that in his opinion, this was further confirmation of the association of this condition with the 'iniquities' of urban living.[125]

At Holloway specific information regarding GPI may have been omitted from patient notes in order to spare patients' families. But, during Holloway's first eighteen months, several known cases of the disease were admitted, two of which were women. GPI was held to be responsible for five out of the seven deaths recorded during that period.[126] In 1890, the numbers were sufficiently problematic to prompt Rees Philipps to state his conviction that as many as one-quarter of all male admissions were GPI sufferers, which adversely affected the death rate for male patients. He observed that, although women were more likely to suffer from insanity in general, they were more likely to be cured and they were not usually diagnosed with general paralysis. He explained:

> The nervous organisation of the female is less stable than that of the male, and is therefore more liable to merely functional disturbance, while in the male the nervous centres, though more stable, are also more prone to serious organic lesions, such as general paralysis, from which the female is comparatively exempt.[127]

It is perhaps indicative of the confusing range of symptoms associated with GPI that the Holloway doctors failed to make the connection between a husband and wife who were simultaneously undergoing treatment for GPI.[128]

Despite the problem of GPI, overall, Holloway's recovery rates were higher than those of Brookwood; in 1889, for example, they stood at nearly 40 per cent for certified patients (41 per cent for boarders). Death rates that year stood at 13 per cent, two-thirds of which were male. In common with his Brookwood counterpart, Rees Philipps was emphatic that early admission and treatment were crucial for recovery, and in 1890 he proudly announced a 100 per cent recovery rate for twenty-four cases of acute mania, precisely because they had been admitted to Holloway whilst in the early stages of their disease. He pointed out that their recovery had also been facilitated by the use of 'the continuous warm bath, which in carefully selected cases proved to be a therapeutic agent of great value'.[129] Holloway Sanatorium frequently measured itself against the performance of other institutions, cited here by Holloway, as private asylums, when some in fact were charitable institutions that received charitable patients. In

1892, the superintendent was delighted to report that they were second only to St Andrew's Hospital Northampton in the 'league table', as seen in Table 5.2.[130]

Table 5.2: Recovery rates for private asylums in 1892.

Recovery rates 1892	(per cent)
Holloway Sanatorium	54.3
Bethlem	48.9
Royal Manchester Hospital	48.7
St Andrew's Hospital	69.1
St Luke's	45.3
Barnwood House	40.0

Source: Holloway Annual Report 1893.

Conclusion

Brookwood Asylum and Holloway Sanatorium aimed to contain, care for and ultimately 'cure' their patients, so that they were sufficiently recovered or relieved of symptoms and were well enough to live safely outside the asylum walls. Their patients suffered from the same primary illnesses which could often be attended by additional complications such as epilepsy or GPI that reduced the possibility of making a full recovery. Some illnesses were more commonly associated with both sexes at Brookwood and Holloway. The known causes of insanity also showed some commonalities between the two patient groups, although some variations have been shown, such as the association between insanity and social deprivation being more prevalent amongst Brookwood patients, and also that intemperance was attributed to fewer Holloway patients.

Recovery and death rates were closely monitored and seen as indicators of efficacy and success. Both institutions operated a therapeutics policy that encompassed all aspects of moral therapy which managed every aspect of the patient's life, from their physical environment, their diet, to exercise and spiritual guidance. This did not prevent the inclusion of other therapeutic methods producing a somewhat eclectic mix of treatment. At Holloway Sanatorium, patients and families expected very high standards, and the management incorporated new facilities and treatments wherever possible. The sanatorium's independent status offered more opportunities to provide varied and intense therapeutic regimes that included a wider range of moral and physical treatments. The latest available drugs were used more widely, while at Brookwood these were restricted for financial reasons and quickly discontinued when seen to be ineffective. Increasingly, the large numbers of admissions, the seeming incurability of many and a growing belief in the importance of hereditary predispositions to insanity, provided the rationale for minimal chemical intervention.

Despite this, the Brookwood doctors experimented by carrying out the relatively rare procedure of trepanning when other therapies appeared to have failed. Chemical intervention was limited to the more violent cases as well as those who were actively suicidal. The superintendent attempted a particularly humane type of seclusion whenever possible, which was applauded by other experts in the field of psychological medicine. This was indicative of the asylum's efforts at humane management and its concern to provide the best treatment possible for patients with some chance of recovery. At Holloway, gymnastics, massage and Turkish baths were used as therapeutic interventions that were not available for the Brookwood patients. Electric therapy, whilst not exclusive to the sanatorium, was more likely to be put to use there than at Brookwood.

There was also an impressive schedule of entertainments at Holloway; partly this would have been expected by the patients' families, but also the management was less likely to use work therapy to physically exhaust and distract the patients. Brookwood's tightly organized work schedules were not the only way patients were kept occupied as a number of varied amusements and facilities were also available, despite budgetary restrictions and the larger numbers of inmates. Both Brookwood and Holloway adhered to certain contemporary class delineations in the diagnoses of their patients, their approach to therapeutics and care, and their expectations of appropriate social behaviour. Despite the many apparent advantages of being incarcerated at Holloway, there were some serious incidences of neglect and incompetence that were not seen at Brookwood. The Weir case was famous in this regard, but there were also a number of notable suicides that occurred within the sanatorium and these are examined in the next chapter.

6 SUICIDE, SELF-HARM AND MADNESS IN THE ASYLUM

Introduction

Despite an enduring academic interest in suicide, there has been little systematic research on the role that individual asylums have played in public responses to the phenomenon. This is in spite of the fact that 'suicidal' patients formed a central component in lay and professional identification of insanity, in the reasons for committal and subsequent treatment and, though arguably to a lesser degree, the therapeutic milieu of the institutions. Case studies of asylums have revealed the stories of individual patients confined within private licensed homes, charitable lunatic hospitals, and county and borough asylums, and recent work on the history of clinical psychiatry has explored the conceptual relationship between suicidal intention and the classification of insanity.[1] There has been little research on how communities identified suicidal intentions and attempts as demonstrating insanity, and how asylums were used to control and provide surveillance over those who had attempted to take their own lives. Recently, the work of Sarah York and other scholars have begun to address these issues.[2]

While suicide has not been entirely ignored in the historiography of psychiatry, prior to the 1980s there were few detailed studies of suicide in England.[3] Recently, pioneering monographs have formed the basis of a discipline that seeks to remove the subject from the margins of medical and social history. For example, Michael MacDonald and Terrance Murphy have illustrated the secularization of suicide during early modern England.[4] They have demonstrated that suicide itself had a social and cultural history embedded in the changing context of pre-industrial and early industrial society. Over the course of the first half of the nineteenth century, there was a perceptible shift from regarding suicide as predominantly a lay, religious and legal concern, to one in which medical men had a role to play.[5] As Olive Anderson pointed out in her seminal work on suicide in Victorian and Edwardian England, this reconfiguration of suicide as being symptomatic of mental illness benefited many agencies. Medical superintendents of asylums regarded the inclusion of the suicidally inclined as an important constituency of clients. Such alienists postulated the belief that suicide could be controlled if the appropriate action were taken early enough. This, they argued, was best achieved by way of institutional care and control.[6] Anderson's work reinforces the impression given by the Commissioners in Lunacy in 1882 that the asylum was an effective force in the prevention of suicide and the supervision of the suicidal.[7]

Barbara Gates's work on Victorian suicide presents a social survey of suicide and contemporary attitudes to self-murder, asserting that, as the century progressed, the Victorians regarded the act with more compassion and understanding.[8] However, Gates disregards attempts at prevention, treatment or the dilemmas faced by the medical profession when confronted with the most overt acts of self-harm. Whilst not writing directly on the subject of suicide, the medicalization of suicidal behaviour was a key theme in the work of Pat Jalland.[9] With the absorption of bourgeois values by the early Victorian middle classes, she argued that suicidal deaths became inextricably associated with contemporary notions of 'bad deaths', and were an affront to both civilized society and religious beliefs. Accordingly, while a coroner's verdict of death by (suicidal) insanity carried with it the stigma of lunacy, it at least guaranteed a Christian burial which afforded some comfort for grieving relatives.[10]

Research on suicide in England has begun to challenge Durkheim's well-known pronouncements on the relationship between industrialization and suicide.[11] The perceived connection between urban life and suicide has been mooted since the seventeenth century.[12] Durkheim's basic principle was that the rapid social changes that occurred in the nineteenth century and which were accompanied by migration and urbanization, proved detrimental to the social fabric of society. This produced demoralization, psychological dislocation and increased suicides. Anderson has argued that there is insufficient empirical data to support the contention that suicide rates in towns were any higher than those found in rural areas. Conversely, MacDonald's data illustrates a decline in suicide rates towards the latter half of the eighteenth century, the very time when the industrial revolution was gathering momentum, when, he also argues, there was a marked increase in the accurate reportage of suicides, partly due the increased secularization of self-murder. In his insightful case study of nineteenth-century Hull, Victor Bailey asserts his belief that Durkheim's basic dictums need to be 'substantially' revised in any empirical study of suicide.[13]

Bailey's work continued the tradition of researching suicide by way of death certificates, coroner's reports and official statistics. This ensured a wide coverage of those who completed the act, but necessarily ignores those who failed in attempts to end their lives. Attempted suicide has remained a largely unexplored dimension of the history of psychiatry, with the exception of Anderson, who considers the role of medical men in suicide prevention. Although suicidal patients have been detailed in individual case studies in the histories of various mental institutions, there were no specific accounts devoted to the asylums' response to suicidality.[14] However, a body of work is slowly emerging which seeks to address this and which focuses specifically on the relationship between non-restraint and surveillance in the care of the suicidal patients.[15] The recent work of Sarah York considers the nature and extent of surveillance as an effective tool in the management of suicide prevention and she has highlighted the importance of the attendants in implementing the practical aspects of suicide prevention.[16]

Suicide, and the threat of suicide, were important criteria in the determination and classification of insanity for all parties who sought institutional confinement, be they official agencies, medical practitioners or relatives. As excerpts from the Brookwood and Holloway records show, suicidal predisposition included a wide range of intentions and behaviours, from those who had clearly and violently attempted self-murder, to melancholics who expressed a vague wish to die, or who refused to eat. At both asylums, there were similarities in the management and treatment of the allegedly suicidal, but there were also differences that can be partially explained by the class perceptions and the suitability of some preventative measures. As the use of mechanical restraint declined, staff were instructed to employ a range of strategic measures that included surveillance, seclusion, protective clothing and force-feeding. As patient numbers rose, there was a corresponding increase in the use of narcotics and sedatives to protect patients at risk and, arguably, to aid asylum management.

Suicide and the Asylum in Nineteenth-Century England

In 1882 the Commissioners in Lunacy launched a special investigation into the prevalence of suicidal lunatics admitted to licensed homes, mental hospitals and county asylums. Aggregating returns from individual institutions from the previous two years, the Commissioners estimated that 3,877 (29 per cent) of asylum admissions were allegedly 'suicidal', representing 27 per cent of all male admissions, and nearly a third (30 per cent) of female admissions. Bearing in mind that 76,765 lunatics were institutionally confined during part or all of that year, the Commissioners observed that only seventeen patients had taken their own lives. They concluded that this was due to the high levels of institutional 'care and attention which [have been] bestowed on suicidal patients'.[17]

Other commentators were more conservative. George Savage, himself a medical superintendent, admitted that he did not believe that 'more than five per cent' of admissions were 'actively suicidal', which he defined as those 'patients who have made serious attempts on their lives, and [were] likely to repeat them'.[18]

Even accepting his more restrictive definition, fewer than two dozen patients out of approximately 500 'actively suicidal' patients 'successfully' took their lives in licensed institutions, compared to over a thousand suicides for England and Wales during the same year. The suicide statistics gathered by the national inspectorate indicated the apparent success of asylum doctors and the increasing willingness of communities to use asylums to control the suicidal poor.

After the 1862 Lunatics Property Act, medical superintendents were required to alert coroners of any institutional deaths.[19] Detailed reports of suspicious deaths and suicides were also sent to the Commissioners in Lunacy. The death of an inmate by suicide was seen as a blight on the good running of the institution and was as damning, by this time, as the use of mechanical restraint. Inquests were often held and negligent attendants brought to account. The 1882 investigation of the Commissioners in Lunacy reflected the heightened professional interest in the plight of suicidal individuals throughout England and Wales. Partially as a result of their report, medical superintendents like Savage, coroners such as Wynn Westcott, and physicians such as Henry Morselli[20] wrote extensively about suicide and its prevention in the early and mid-1880s, nearly a decade before Durkheim's famous treatise appeared.[21]

Extending their professional territory to include the suicidal, alienists made their case for institutional treatment by asserting that suicide could be avoided with early intervention. The management of Brookwood and Holloway saw suicidal propensity as an important criterion in the determination and classification of insanity and the decision to seek institutional confinement.[22] The 'statement of particulars' on reception orders included personal details, previous history and other social and medical characteristics as well as any indication of suicidal and/or violent intentions. The recording of these details was an acknowledgement of the connection between madness and self-murder.

The examination of patient characteristics in these two asylums shows that patients were labelled suicidal for many reasons, and that the medical practitioners had some understanding of the relationship between specific disordered mental states and suicidal behaviour and intentions. The policies adopted by the respective superintendents of Brookwood and Holloway towards the threat of suicide were remarkably similar. The asylum records enable the consideration of the social construction of suicidal behaviour, and are a useful comparison to the more frequently used coroners' reports, which underpin most historical reconstructions of research on Victorian suicide. As York has pointed out, asylum histories usually only discussed suicide prevention in relation to the growth of the non-restraint movement, which, although relevant, adds little to understanding how individual institutions dealt with these inmates.[23] The York Retreat, Norfolk Asylum and the Littlemore Asylum, Oxford, all used seclusion to manage excitable or epileptic patients, but not for those who were suicidal;

for these cases, surveillance remained the primary intervention.[24] MacKenzie's study of Ticehurst Asylum showed how the medical superintendent, Dr Hayes Newington, prioritized suicide prevention because of its adverse effect on the welfare and morale of patients and staff. Brushfield and Rees Philipps expressed similar opinions that were fuelled by their concern at the rising number of allegedly suicidal admissions to their institutions.

Throughout the first half of the nineteenth century, asylums received many patients who had recently attempted or threatened self-murder. By the time of the 1845 legislation, medical superintendents were familiar with the difficulties associated with suicidal lunatics; Parry-Jones, for instance, showed that private madhouse keepers often accepted such patients sent by families and parishes.[25] Similarly, Digby acknowledged that straitjackets were commonly used at the York Retreat in the 1820s, when patients were feared to be in danger of killing themselves.[26] Brookwood and Holloway reflect this intersection of institutional medical practice and suicidal behaviour. They drew their patient populations from different social and geographical backgrounds which provide opportunities to consider the impact class and gender made upon nosology and therapeutics.

Suicide and Psychiatry

Forbes Winslow, in one of the first works specifically devoted to the subject (1840), remarked that suicide had been viewed as the 'theme of the novel and of the drama', as either a mortal sin or a heroic option.[27] Gradually, this gave way to a perception of suicide as a manifestation of irrational behaviour that should be addressed by the medical profession.[28] Medical treatises on mental illness began to discuss aspects of suicidal propensity and the signs leading to a diagnosis of temporary insanity. Debates covered spontaneous suicide, the pathogenesis of suicidal impulse, the identification of those most at risk, the timeliness of intervention, and the most appropriate treatment.

Psychiatric writings claimed that suicide could be successfully prevented by timely and specialist intervention. In 1830, John Conolly highlighted the dangers of overlooking the potentially suicidal, the unhappy or 'irritable' personalities, and the implications of disregarding their insanity until it was too late:

> At the moment of suicide, some impression becomes intolerable which was not considered intolerable before, or which, if the suicide was prevented, would not be considered intolerable the day after. A distracted man cuts his throat while he is dressing: if we could arrest his hand, and seat him at the dinner table with his friends, he would look back upon the frenzy of the previous hour with as much concern as the passionate man looks back on the imprecations and stamping of his angry fit. He would now attend more calmly to the cause of the disagreeable emotion, and compare it with many alleviations he would find he possessed. He would consider the act of self-murder, and start from it with horror. He dies because he cannot attend to

all these circumstances, and because, therefore, he makes no comparison. The loss of comparison is madness, and in his madness he destroys himself.[29]

Forbes Winslow further advocated that the successful treatment of suicide depended on strict attention being paid 'to those apparently trifling alterations of temper and disposition, those deviations from the usual mode of thinking and acting'.[30] As early as 1809, John Haslam indicated the association between melancholia and suicidal predisposition. To minimize risk, he advocated the patient's isolation from the familiar environment – and the family – as being vital for their well-being.[31] For some cases, visitors were beneficial, but they could also prove a dangerous stimulant, particularly if they were unaware of the patient's true condition:

> ignorant people often, after a few minutes conversation with the patient, will suppose him perfectly recovered, and acquaint him with their opinion; this induces him to suppose that he is well, and he frequently becomes impatient of confinement and restraint. From such improper intercourse I have known many patients relapse, and in two instances I have a well-founded suspicion that it excited attempts at suicide.[32]

Brushfield frequently highlighted the high numbers of suicidal Brookwood admissions to the Committee of Visitors and the Commissioners in Lunacy. He emphasized the difficulties of caring for these patients. He, too, firmly postulated the link between melancholia and suicide, echoing Forbes Winslow, who stated in his 1840 treatise on suicide: 'There is no more frequent cause of suicide than visceral derangement, leading to melancholia and hypochondria'.[33] In 1880, Brushfield defined two types of suicidal patients. First, there were those who had no obvious suicidal motive but who persistently endangered their lives, and so were described as suicidal on their certificates. The second group were patients who were focused on self-destruction as a result of their illness.[34] The first group was typified by patients who refused food, whether or not this was due to 'complete indifference, from the idea that it is poisoned, from the belief that it has been obtained by depriving others etc.'.[35] The second group constituted a much more serious threat:

> I would urge upon all medical practitioners the necessity of regarding all cases of melancholia as having a suicidal tendency, whether or not there have been threats or attempts indicating it; the depressing nature of the symptoms, if it does not manifest itself at first, always tends to develop. The medical man should make the relatives understand this, especially if they are averse to sending the patient away from home to be treated.[36]

Throughout the century, suicidal propensity continued to be associated with melancholia. Westcott linked it to fifty-seven cases of melancholia, as opposed to twenty-one cases of mania, sixteen of ordinary dementia, fifteen of senile dementia and eight of idiocy. He also asserted that 'the proportion of suicidal tendency was higher among pauper than among well-to-do lunatics'.[37] Marriage offered no protection against suicide, he noted: 'marriage 32, celibacy 24, and widowhood 29, and of married persons, more females than males'.[38] Scull has argued that the inclusion of melancholy and its 'plethora of disguises'[39] which included suicidal tendency, was part of the increased language of insanity that helped swell the numbers of those considered insane.[40]

John Bucknill and Daniel Hack Tuke, authors of the standard Victorian textbook on psychological medicine, proposed that attempted suicide whilst insane, whether temporary or not, occurred in three conditions associated with states of unsound mind. They described these as 'monomania', where the patient was inclined to self-destruction; 'melancholia', when the sufferer was driven to despair; and, lastly, 'delusional', when voices instructed the patient to self-harm.[41] The medical profession drew its information not only from the patients under its control, but also from the statistics published from coroners' reports, with their tables of regional and sex variations in suicide mortality. These data on 'completed' suicide endorsed the view that more men 'successfully' committed suicide, a confirmation of the pressures that they endured and which drove them to such desperate action. It might have been expected that women were potentially more vulnerable to suicide, on account of biological changes throughout their lives that could lead to depression. But the view was that women were not necessarily less suicidally inclined, but that they were allegedly less competent at carrying it out. As Henry Morselli stated: 'the sexual difference in suicide would cause the supposition that a certain strength of character and moral force, which is generally wanting in the woman, is necessary'.[42]

Such notions about gender differences endured; Havelock Ellis believed that it was the messiness of the most effective methods that caused women's squeamishness; if the body could simply disappear in the process, then more women would attempt the act.[43] As the numbers of city dwellers swelled, so too were traditional views on women challenged, a process described by Kushner as 'gender chaos' that was closely associated with vice and modernity. Women, by entering an urbanized workforce were, in effect, acting like men, and so endangered themselves and the family, the cornerstone of society. This concern with women's role in society, Kushner believed, was at the very heart of those contemporary concerns of urbanization and suicide.[44]

Table 6.1: Suicides in England and Wales, 1861–70.

Province	Actual number male	Actual number female	Male suicides per 1,000f.
London	1,909	760	2,512
South-eastern counties	1,284	378	3,396
South-Midland counties	628	212	2,962
Eastern counties	530	176	3,011
South-western counties	762	297	2,565

Province	Actual number male	Actual number female	Male suicides per 1,000f.
West-Midland counties	1,083	357	3,033
North-Midland	742	295	2,515
North-western	1,555	500	3,111
Yorkshire	970	403	2,406
Northern counties	528	202	2,618
Monmouthshire and Wales	311	127	2,448

Source: H. Morselli, *Suicide, an Essay on Comparative Moral Statistics* (London: C. Kegan Paul Co., 1881), p. 193.

The association between city life and suicide was long-established, with roots traceable to the seventeenth century.[45] It gained momentum with industrialization, fuelled by middle-class preoccupations with the unpredictability of a new urbanized working class, who were becoming 'civilized' and educated, but were unequipped to deal with it; the 'threat' of upward social mobility. Writing in 1840, Forbes Winslow summed up the dangers: 'There cannot be a doubt, but that the general diffusion of knowledge, and the desire to place within the command of the humblest person the advantages of education, have not a little tended to promote the crime of suicide'.[46]

Westcott and Morselli believed that more suicides occurred in towns and cities than in the countryside, partly due to the intense struggle for survival, increased pressures on daily life as well as the perceived steep moral decline that occurred in cities. Both Morselli and Masaryk's influential texts covered the supposed epidemic of suicide, which they viewed as the disease of civilized nations.[47] S. A. K. Strachen's 1893 publication, *On Suicide and Insanity: A Philosophical and Sociological Study*, reflected an almost universal belief in the associations between modern city life and suicidal impulse, and Durkheim's later work developed the argument that suicide was a social problem as opposed to a moral crime.

Suicidal Admissions to Brookwood and Holloway

Morselli's speculation on completed suicide, and on the male–female balance, is refuted by an analysis of the returns of those admitted to Brookwood. Over a third (34 per cent) of all Brookwood admissions was classified as suicidal. Women dominated the suicidally predisposed, covering 62 per cent of female admissions, as opposed to 38 per cent of males.[48] Taking 1871–81 as an example, nearly one-third of all first admissions were classified as suicidal, and women accounted for over 60 per cent of these.[49] In 1879, Brushfield stated that just over 48 per cent of inmates had suicidal propensities, comprising 349 females and 137 males. Nearly one-third of the 1878 admissions were certified as being suicidal and over half of these had made an actual attempt on their lives prior to admission.[50] He could not foresee that the problem would decrease. Women listed as suicidal correspond roughly to the age-class of all female admissions, whereas men's likelihood to be listed as suicidal rose dramatically after the age of fifty, largely the result of unemployment, attendant poverty and lack of prospects. Married men and single women also feature disproportionately, relative to their representation in the admissions at Surrey County Asylum.

As for Morselli's contention that urban life created situations which fostered suicidality, an evaluation of the remaining cases in Brookwood on 14 April 1875 by union, showed that – of a total of forty-seven patients – just under one-third were suicidal, and most of these (60 per cent) originated from the metropolitan unions.[51] Holloway's incomplete records and irregular recording does not enable a direct comparison. The suicidal ideation was not recorded in the admission registers and not all documentation has survived. The individual case notes show that many patients were of a suicidal disposition, self-harming or regularly attempting suicide while in the sanatorium, using whatever (limited) means were available to them. Stella S. was admitted at the age of twenty in August 1902, just two months after delivering a healthy baby girl. Delusional and depressed, she had hinted at suicide, but had not attempted it. Whilst in the sanatorium, she refused food and spoke repeatedly of wishing to die. She began to pull out her hair and was often restrained by a 'strong dress'. Over the next few months, she tried to strangle herself with her belt, and later with the chain from the bath plug.[52]

Writing in 1885, Wynn Westcott, Deputy Coroner for Central Middlesex, marvelled at the small number of the means of suicide that were selected, when there were so many possibilities (see Table 6.2). His investigations also revealed distinct differences between the sexes in their chosen methodology. The same year, William Ogle presented a paper to the Royal Statistical Society on mortality and occupation in England and Wales, some of which was devoted to suicidal mortality. Reaching the same conclusions, he noted that both men and women had favoured four means of killing themselves, namely hanging, throat cutting, drowning and self-poisoning. The patterns of reported suicide showed that women preferred drowning and poisoning: 'The female sex is the especial patroness of death by drowning in every country; twice as many women as men drown themselves in Europe every year'.[53]

Men, by contrast, usually resorted to hanging, a pattern repeated throughout England and Europe. The second most significant method was cutting their own throats, popular in England and Ireland, but rarely found elsewhere. By contrast, 'Opening the veins is an almost forgotten practice'.[54] Self-poisoning was apparently very popular in England and the United States, and, not surprisingly, opium, morphia and their preparations were the most frequently used, as well-known poisons, rather than an overdose of 'safe' drugs, was preferred. Other everyday and easily procured poisons included prussic acid, cyanide of potassium (used in photography) carbolic acid and derivatives used for disinfecting, essential oil of bitter almonds (cookery), and anti-vermin preparations such as strychnine.[55] Within the asylums, it was the popularity and relative ease of hanging, both in attempted and completed suicides, which posed the greatest challenge. Although not conclusive, the admission records and contemporary accounts of completed suicides endorse the view that women generally employed less violent means of suicide.

Suicide methods calculated by two contemporary observers are shown below. 'Other causes', as defined by Westcott, included jumping under rail/vehicles, or from heights, strangling, cuts and stabs, burns, scalds and explosions, and suffocation by vapours. Ogle's were similar, but he included cuts and stabs with the 'cut throat' group.

Table 6.2: Method of suicides in England and Wales, *c.* 1881, as calculated by two contemporary observers.[56]

Means	Percentage of males		Percentage of females	
	Ogle	Wescott	Ogle	Wescott
Hanging	41.7	34.3	24.0	23.1
Cut throat	20.7	18.6	12.9	11.6
Drowning	15.2	17.5	26.4	35.2
Poison	7.9	9.0	14.5	19.2
Fire-arms	6.7	8.2	1.0	0.6
All other causes	7.3	12.4	21.2	10.2

Multiple suicide attempts often involved several methods. Before his incarceration in Brookwood, Alfred L., a 36-year-old married labourer from Lambeth, had made two attempts. On the first occasion, he tried to drown himself, and on the second, he cut his throat, which resulted in permanent damage that made swallowing difficult.[57] As many Brookwood patients came from the workhouses, accompanying details were often minimal, although some patients revealed a suicidal disposition shortly after arrival. Violent and extreme patients were removed as quickly as possible to the asylum from the workhouses. George L. was sent from the Dorking Workhouse infirmary to Brookwood on 12 February 1877. A tailor by trade, this 56-year-old married man with melancholia had only been in the workhouse a short time before he amputated his penis with a pair of scissors. With only six members of staff (including the workhouse master and his wife), and up to 250 inmates at any one time, it was decided that the asylum was the only place where he could be properly cared for.[58]

The high numbers of suicidal admissions to Brookwood should be viewed with a degree of scepticism, as workhouses used the description to be rid of their most troublesome and disruptive inmates.[59] 'Suicidal' covered many different types of behaviour, and failed to distinguish between self-harming and suicidal behaviour. Both were seen as evidence of insanity and loss of self-control, however temporary. Food refusal was regarded as a self-destructive behaviour, or at the very least, was indicative of a patient lacking the will to live. Self-mutilation was relatively rare in asylums (although it did occur), and together with other 'indirect' forms of self-inflicted bodily damage, was usually considered by both institutions as indicating suicidal intent. There was little recognition at this time that the self-harmer did not necessarily seek death. However, the inclusion of most types of self-harm as suggestive of suicidal intent was in keeping with later research that confirmed self-harm was a risk factor in attempted suicide.[60] Self-harming behaviours that were categorized by alienists in later medical texts ranged from 'major' damage that included amputation, castration and oedipism (self-damage to the eyes), to those of a more 'minor' type that included 'hair-plucking and face-picking'.[61]

Opportunities for suicide after admission were limited, so that self-strangulation and hanging were the easiest to attempt. Ellen A., aged forty-two, arrived at Brookwood in July 1879, after spending seven years in Caterham Asylum where 'she was discharged from there 2 days ago as unfit on account of her frequent attempts to commit suicide'.[62] She was treated at Newington Infirmary after her last effort before her move to Brookwood. Six days later, she attempted suicide by self-strangulation. Transferred a few months later to another institution, she was returned to Brookwood in late 1881, and on two occasions within a five-month period attempted to strangle herself, firstly with the laces of her stays, and secondly with her apron strings.[63] Belts and sheets were other everyday items that were used by patients for such purposes; yet others tried to jump through windows, either at the asylum or during transportation from the workhouse or home.

In 1892, despite all precautions, Brookwood suffered two completed male suicides, both by hanging. The first, 'D. W.', had been admitted suffering from melancholia with suicidal tendencies, but six weeks after his admission he was believed to have recovered sufficiently so as to no longer warrant special observation. He had continued to slowly improve but nearly one year after his admission, he went missing after evening exercise in the airing court. Shortly afterwards, he was discovered suspended from a tree.[64] Benjamin S. was admitted from his home in Petersham, Surrey, in October 1892. He was suffering from mania, and had threatened to destroy himself, his wife and his children. Following his admission, he also began to gradually improve and worked cleaning the wards. However, he retained some of his original delusions, and on the morning of 1 May 1893, he took his own life. Reporting on the same day, to the Commissioners in Lunacy, James Barton (medical superintendent) wrote:

> I beg to report for the information of the Commissioners in Lunacy, that this patient who was admitted from the Richmond Union on October 29th last, committed sui-

cide this morning at 8.15 by hanging himself with a piece of box rope in one of the ward closets.

When admitted, he was suffering from 'Mania with delusions', and was stated to have threatened suicide. He was at intervals depressed and lachrymose but was however not considered actively suicidal. He has slept under continuous supervision at night although he has been regularly employed in various ways. He did not exhibit any mental improvement.

He was spoken to at 8.5 am. today when employed in ward cleaning, by one of the attendants who asked him how he was and he replied 'the same as usual' and at 8.10 am. he was noticed by another attendant. Neither of these observed anything unusual in his manner.

At 8.15 am. one of the ward patients on going into the W.C. found him suspended by the neck the body being in a sitting position and slightly raised off the ground, the rope being tied to an upright near the window about 5ft. 6in. from the ground.

The patient immediately summoned the attendants who ran in and cut the rope and at once resorted to artificial respiration, but on Dr Gayton's arrival life was found to be extinct.

I have carefully considered all the circumstances of this case and conclude that the suicide was the result of sudden impulse and cannot attach any blame to any one of the Ward Attendants.'[65]

At the inquest held at the asylum two days later, the coroner declared that 'The Deceased at the time of hanging himself was of unsound state of mind'.[66] The asylum and the attendants were exonerated of all blame, although how Benjamin S. obtained the rope was not clarified. There is little evidence that attendants were blamed for such deaths (unlike the strict discipline that was enforced when charges of unnecessary abuse or violence were proven) which suggests that the difficulties in keeping patients safe were widely recognized. Guidance on caring for the suicidal was provided in contemporary handbooks; the cornerstone was constant surveillance, and it was recommended that the patients' clothing and bedding were regularly checked for any hidden and dangerous objects.[67]

Dr Brushfield's experiences led him to believe that, whilst methods of self-destruction varied greatly, if a patient was sufficiently determined, he or she would seize any and every opportunity to end their lives. He gave the history of one particularly resolute man who came under his care and who was later discharged from Brookwood as recovered:

The patient first threw himself under the wheels of a cab, and was run over and most severely bruised; he then sat down on a fire; next he jumped from a three storey window; he tried to strangle himself with a sheet; he swallowed a bottleful of soap and opium liniment; finally, after his removal to the workhouse, he inflicted a severe wound in his throat, and in this condition he was received into the asylum.[68]

Although Holloway records are incomplete, there appear to have been fewer declared suicidal patients admitted, although this is open to doubt. The available data showed that nearly a third of Holloway's admissions were diagnosed as suffering from melancholia which, as noted, was associated with suicidal propensity. Families may have hidden the shame of such inclinations, so that the information was not available at the time of admission. The numbers of melancholic admissions to Holloway continued to rise, leading the acting superintendent in 1899 to comment that this 'disease' outstripped mania as the main illness in the sanatorium. This he partially attributed to influenza epidemics which lowered the spirits and increased vulnerability.[69]

Like Brushfield, Rees Philipps associated melancholia with self-destruction, stating that melancholic patients were often subject to the most 'desperately suicidal tendencies'. Food refusal was viewed as indicative of suicidal intent and its prevalence at Holloway meant that labour and time-intensive force-feeding was part of the daily routine. A year free from suicide, or indeed any serious attempt at self-harm, was reported with cautious relief, although Rees Philipps felt that 'this freedom from suicide is not always a matter for congratulation'.[70] Constant surveillance was viewed by the medical profession as the only effective method of suicide prevention, yet he personally viewed the strategy as an infringement of patient privacy. Given the middle- and upper-class origins of the Holloway patients, Rees Philipps was particularly conscious of such sensitivities. Further, he believed that surveillance could actually stimulate a patient's suicidal propensity. In this, his view echoed that of Henry Savage, who commented, after years of observing suicidal patients (mainly from his private practice):

> Patients have repeatedly told me that when constantly watched they felt as if they were being dared to do a thing, and naturally set themselves to evade their tormentors. A perfect attendant does not irritate a patient perhaps, but I have not found one yet.[71]

Bemoaning the limited number of preventative measures available, Philipps radically stated that 'suicidal accidents must and will occur, and if they do not occur occasionally, the suspicion arises that supervision is too strict'.[72] As evidence, he commented that, in Scotland, suicides were seen and recorded as accidents and no blame attached to the medical staff:

> If a Superintendent looks to the spirit of the rules, and, in spite of some risk, labours for the greatest amount of benefit for his patients as a whole, he is sympathised with in any failure, and encouraged in his work.[73]

This view was not shared by Brookwood's management. Accountability and class perceptions may have been contributory factors, but interestingly, even at the private asylum of Ticehurst, there was no apparent endorsement of Savage's view, and patients believed to be suicidal were never left alone.[74] Rees Philipp's approach, from which he never wavered, must have been acceptable to the committee, reflected perhaps by the often brief references to 'accidents' or attempted self-harm which were almost seen as inevitable. In the superintendent's annual report, he commented that 'One lady succeeded in setting fire to her night-dress, but though she sustained extensive superficial burns, finally made a good recovery'.[75] In 1892, it was briefly recorded that 'The close of the year was marred by the death of a lady, who on Boxing Day drank some carbolic acid which had been carelessly left on the washstand in a nurse's room'.[76] There may have also been a strong wish to 'play-down' such incidents as these could have detracted from the impression of the sanatorium as a safe custodial haven for the middle-class insane.

Despite Rees Philipp's views, some patients were so violent in their suicide attempts that drastic measures were taken to prevent their ultimate destruction. Edith R. began her lengthy stay at Holloway in July 1886 at the age of thirty-seven. This unmarried woman had a history of trying to poison herself and others with strychnine, which had led to her incarceration at the Warneford Asylum (Oxford) before she arrived at the sanatorium. On her first day, she seized at a pair of scissors to harm herself, as well as tying a sheet around her neck later that evening. Throughout her stay, she remained excitable, smashed ornaments and attacked patients and staff. She banged her head repeatedly against the walls, tore at her face and tried to swallow hairpins. (Thereafter no nurse in her gallery was allowed to wear any pins of any kind.)

She was observed to have entered a period of dementia accompanied by intense mania that was so severe that she often had to be placed in the padded room for most of the night, where she was visited by a nurse every quarter of an hour.[77] She was treated with several compounds and hypodermic injections of drugs that included potassium bromide and the addictive paraldehyde and chloral hydrate. She was often restrained in a jacket and gloves, and surveillance was strictly maintained at all times as she 'will swallow pins or pieces of broken glass and is very dangerous to others unless extremely carefully watched'.[78]

Rose C. was admitted to Holloway Sanatorium, first as a voluntary boarder in 1891 and again in 1893 as a certified patient. An unmarried woman, she was 'discharged' a year later but remained at the sanatorium until 1901 as a 50-year-old voluntary boarder. On 14 October that year, she went to visit her relations, but returned dazed and confused on 26 October. She soon began to exhibit self-destructive and suicidal behaviour. On 1 November, she drank a bottle of eau de cologne and was treated in the infirmary. One week later, she tried to swallow her artificial teeth, rammed them down her throat and then attempted to drown herself in the bath. By 13 November, she was certified, and a suicide caution note issued so that she was under constant surveillance.[79] Voluntary boarders with suicidal propensity did not always remain at Holloway for their treatment after certification; this could be due to inability to pay, and not being accepted under charitable status (suicidality did not mean automatic acceptance by the board) or because patients' families chose alternative hospitals. Margaret O. was a voluntary boarder from 24 July 1893. Melancholic apparently as a result of a failed love affair, she had tried to self-poison the day before she arrived at the sanatorium. She made little improvement during her stay and, by the end of November, was certified and sent to Exeter County Asylum, but not before she tried to throw herself under a train.[80]

Families were anxious to find the best place for self-destructive relatives but this did not necessarily mean that they wholly subscribed to a 'medical model', or that they saw attempted suicide as a medical problem. As Rab Houston has pointed out, the increased interest in suicide did not necessarily indicate a total medicalization of suicide, which was an uneven, patchy process that did not evolve till after the mid-nineteenth century and which has remained contested.[81] However, many families did choose the asylums as the best place to keep their relatives safe. The husband of Mary Ann sent a letter accompanying her admission to Brookwood on 13 May 1878. He described the circumstances which he saw as bringing about her mental instability and which he hoped would be helpful to the authorities. Their social position had gradually diminished following the decline of his business over twenty years, she suffered 'severe attacks' of rheumatic fever and bronchitis, and she had sought regular solace in alcohol, so that:

> her manner has been quite at variance with her natural quiet disposition, and on the evening of the 8th instant she appeared depressed, but I did not apprehend that her mind was deranged, but during the brief period of two minutes while I left the room, she cut her throat with a table knife which lay on the supper table.[82]

She stayed only a short time in Brookwood and was discharged as recovered on 3 July the same year.

Treatment and Surveillance of Suicidal Patients

The lunacy reform movement advocated institutional treatment of the insane, citing the therapeutic efficacy of moral treatment that gave individual attention to patients, the practice of non-restraint and the involvement of the patient in daily activities of work, leisure and obedience. Suicidal tendencies were believed to be minimized by traditional familial values, and this was reflected in the asylums' re-enactment as an ideal home as part of the total moral therapy.[83]

As York has identified, the successful implementation of suicidal prevention policies very much depended on the co-operation and diligence of the asylum attendants.[84] However, their efficacy in discharging their duties was compromised by the burgeoning size of the inmate population, particularly in the public sector.[85]

As seen, the Brookwood patient-to-staff ratio stood at 10.5 male patients and 12.6 female patients per attendant, and although some errors still occurred, they were more successful in suicide prevention than at Holloway, which offered almost one-to-one care. As Wynn Westcott observed: 'nothing but a constant and lynx-eyed survey will prevent the self-destruction of a large proportion of lunatics, when they have a wave of suicidal tendency passing over their minds'.[86]

Several similar strategies were employed by Brookwood and Holloway to care for and manage their suicidal patients. These practices were common to most asylums, and began with placing suicidal patients under strict surveillance and in specially equipped rooms. Suicidal patients were kept as far away from doors and windows as possible and generally accommodated on the ground floor of the asylum. Window openings were restricted and some enforced with bars. Bed linen was made of non-tearable material. All sharp objects were removed, and night attendants were instructed to regularly check on the patients, often once an hour. During the day, at-risk patients were closely watched; they were not allowed any sharp objects or cutlery, or allowed out of doors alone. Broadly speaking, vigilant surveillance prevailed, despite some recognition that it could be interpreted as an invasion of privacy and was not necessarily beneficial for all 'suicidal' patients.

At both institutions, surveillance was not always implemented correctly and so occasionally failed. Sometimes, it was unclear as to whether a fatality was an 'accident' or a suicide attempt. Henderson S., a 35-year-old government clerk, suffered from dementia with GPI and arrived at Brookwood on 29 June 1871. His alleged suicidal tendency was questionable, but cannot be wholly discounted. His eleven-month stay at Brookwood had been uneventful until 22 May 1872, when an attendant left a bath of very hot water unattended whilst the patient was nearby. Unobserved, Henderson climbed in and was scalded so badly that he died the following afternoon. The patient's intention was not entirely clear; it may have been attempted suicide but the attendant's negligence was without question. He was subsequently dismissed, and unsurprisingly, the inquest verdict was 'accidental death'. Henderson's case was then successfully absorbed into that regrettable yet acceptable category of accidental deaths, and Brushfield was able to play down the whole incident and protect the reputation of the asylum and his medical staff. In 1878, Brushfield was pleased to report that only two 'successful' suicides had occurred in over eleven years; neither patient had been previously reported as having had suicidal tendencies.[87]

At Holloway, surveillance was viewed as an imperfect method of dealing with potentially suicidal inmates, as discussed above. Rees Philips added that the very size and construction of the Holloway Sanatorium made the likelihood of avoiding all suicides nearly impossible unless surveillance was increased to a level that would almost certainly make the lives of other, non-suicidal, patients unbearable. Francis A., admitted on 24 June 1887, disliked this approach and 'objected strongly to anyone sleeping in her bedroom'; she promptly assaulted the first nurse who attempted to do so.[88]

Rees Philipps emphasized his conviction that constant observation actually hindered recovery. It greatly irritated all patients, but especially the suicidal. Recognizing the directives of the Commissioners in Lunacy, however, he went on to say:

> To sleep or attempt to sleep in an observation dormitory, with a light burning and under a watchful eye, is to many patients a terrible ordeal. But the many must I fear continue to suffer in order that the few may be safe, until such time as different councils prevail with those who direct the treatment of the insane, at any rate in England.[89]

Partially as a result of his reluctance to enforce a policy of the strictest surveillance, Holloway was less effective in preventing suicides or 'accidents'.[90] They were acutely and very publicly embarrassed by the suicide of two patients on the morning of Tuesday, 14 March 1887. James O., aged forty, visited the bathroom at 6 am. But 'during the momentary absence of the keeper, it appears, [he] hung himself with a silk scarf tied to the gas bracket. The deceased lived about an hour after being cut down.'[91] Just two hours later, Eliza S., aged seventy-eight, was found suspended from a rope in the recreation hall. The rope had been left behind by workmen who had erected a platform in the hall, thereby providing the means and opportunity for the unfortunate patient. Eliza S. had not been suspected of being either dangerous or suicidal. At the inquest, Rees Philipps claimed that the only suggestion of her propensity had emerged from a conversation with her son; he had in turn been given this information in a letter received from Dr Langdon Down who had treated her previously as a private patient. He expressed his frustration at the laxity of the lunacy laws that had led to the exclusion of such important information from the deceased's official records. Her behaviour whilst at the sanatorium had given no indication of any suicidal inclinations and she was described as always being quiet and 'appropriate'; on the morning of her death she was neatly dressed and had left her room 'beautifully clean'. On this occasion, the evidence of alleged suicidal propensity, given by a patient's family, was almost disregarded, or at the very least, not accepted by the medical staff. Alternatively, the lack of official notification may have been the ace played by the hospital management in order to escape accusations of blame. The inquest, held at the sanatorium, exonerated the institution from all negligence; the coroner for West Surrey, G. F. Roumieu, commented in his summing up that lunatics 'were very cunning in their methods of making away with themselves', thus reflecting wide-held beliefs regarding the culpability of the insane.[92] The choice of hanging indicated the limited means available to patients intent on suicide and the silk scarf was a resource available to the middle-class Holloway population. The availability of both the scarf and the rope reflect the attitude of the medical staff towards personal freedom, albeit within an institutionalized context.

Both Brookwood and Holloway used chemical restraint to selectively manage the most disruptive and dangerous suicidal cases. Opium, chloral and digitalis were frequently referred to in the case notes of suicidal patients and clinicians often alternated drugs to obtain relief. More unusually, bromide of ammonium and Indian hemp were also administered. Brookwood patient James L., very noisy and allegedly suicidal, was admitted in 1871. He seemed to respond favourably to this combination which had a 'very soothing effect' as opposed to his earlier treatment of opium which had not reduced his noisiness and foul language.[93] Purgatives and shower baths were used, as well as blisters which were applied as counter-irritants to various parts of the body. Catherine H., a 26-year-old hawker, diagnosed with suicidal mania, arrived at Brookwood in June 1871.[94] The asylum used virtually every means at its disposal to manage her. During her four-year stay, she attempted suicide five times, and on the sixth, had hidden a knife inside her clothes that was discovered before any damage occurred. According to her case notes, she was noisy, abusive to the attendants, destructive, obscene, foul-mouthed and filthy. Opium, digitalis, bromide of ammonium with Indian hemp, and cannabis were all tried with variable, though usually short-lived, degrees of success. She was so badly behaved that orders were given to shave her head, clearly as a punishment. Yet, despite this and the application of blisters to the back of her neck, her mania continued virtually unabated and she made further suicide attempts that included setting fire to her dress. The management's apparent dislike of mechanical restraint notwithstanding, it was occasionally used and she was made to wear a strong dress or jacket for a day or two at a time.

Similar preventative measures were used at Holloway, although chemical and physical interventions were more readily applied, given the lack of financial constraint and higher levels of client expectation. Here, treatment often included using electricity in its armoury of defences against those most determined to inflict harm on themselves.[95] Alice M., 'a well-educated housewife of sober habits', was brought to Holloway Sanatorium from Stoke Newington by her husband in June 1886. She suffered from persistent melancholia, allegedly brought about by the menopause and the experience of a 'noisy thoroughfare in Spain'. She would not eat, and had become sullen and dirty. Her husband finally decided upon institutional care after she had squeezed herself through an eighteen-inch window, fallen onto the steps below and sustained severe head wounds. (The implication here is that he had already tried to confine her within the home.) During her first few months in Holloway, she refused to eat and was fed by tube. She constantly threatened self-destruction and one day in November, while unobserved, she tried to poke her eyes out. She was duly restrained in a jacket but still managed to bite her lips and chin so severely that 'She is now a ghastly subject with her lips swollen beyond recognition and eyes the colour of claret'. Throughout her stay, her moods alternated between maniacal excitement, to total withdrawal. Eventually, the medical staff tried electricity, with limited success, though '[it] makes her talk and struggle and during which she sometimes opens her eyes when told to'.[96]

Despite all precautions and treatment, as we have seen, some patients succeeded in taking their own lives whilst in custody. Perhaps one of the most haunting cases was that of Catherine T., who had been transferred from one institution to another. Originally an inmate of Bethlem Hospital for one year, this 32-year-old unmarried nurse, who apparently suffered from melancholia, was removed to Stone Asylum, Buckinghamshire, on 20 July 1870. On 21 April 1871, she was transferred to Springfield Asylum, Wandsworth. She was there only three months before being moved yet again, this time to Brookwood on 14 July. By this time, she was diagnosed as suffering from mania, and her certificate stated that she was 'very suicidally disposed', so that it was thought necessary to restrain her while she was being transferred to Brookwood:

> She was bought in a canvas garment which fitted her person even down to her ankles, the arms however not going through the sleeves, but being folded across her chest close to her skin, the hands being locked in leather gloves. The jacket or whatever it is called being locked at the back by 5 locks. All this complicated arrangement was immediately removed. There was no clothing of ordinary kind under it. The canvas was very thick and rough.[97]

She was generally excitable, but this was exacerbated by any conversation about her time in Wandsworth, an experience that had clearly distressed and frightened her. During the first few weeks at Brookwood, she frequently praised the staff and contrasted her life there to how it had been at Springfield. Initially, she was sufficiently well behaved so as to be granted small privileges such as being allowed to use a sharp knife at meal times. She did so 'without exhibiting any suicidal propensities at present'. She did not, however, sleep well 'owing as she saw it to her great joy at being treated as a human being'. By early 1872, she showed signs of mental deterioration and began to have frequent and seemingly unprovoked violent outbursts where she lashed out at fellow patients and attendants. This became her established pattern of behaviour that was partially managed with doses of morphine and chloral. She made two attempts to escape, once reaching Brookwood Station before being returned by another walking party from the asylum. Early in 1875, she attempted to strangle herself but soon recovered, although her conduct became increasingly unpredictable and extreme. She was once again transferred to Wandsworth Asylum and, within a short time, she committed suicide by hanging.[98]

Catherine was in custodial care when she took her own life, although not in Brookwood. Suicides did sometimes occur after discharge; in 1882 the Commissioners in Lunacy, reporting as it always did on asylum suicides for the previous year, showed that in 1881, three of the twenty-three patients who took their own life, did so out of the asylum. In one particular case, a patient escaped from Whittingham Asylum, lay on the London and North Western Asylum Railway and was found decapitated the next day. Two other patients were judged recovered and had been discharged on probation, but one subsequently shot himself in the head and the other took an overdose of 'chloral'.[99] Clearly, ascertaining someone's fitness to be let out of the asylum 'on trial' was a subjective judgement that sometimes went horribly wrong. After a patient strangled herself with her own bedsheets in 1874 in Morningside Asylum, Hayes Newington, superintendent of the private Ticehurst Asylum, was sufficiently concerned so as to write an article on the 'test for fitness' for discharge, in which he advocated that the 'recognition' by the patient that suicide was wrong should be an important criterion.[100]

At the York Retreat, one patient, having failed to kill herself by cutting her throat, convinced a local youth to buy her a bottle of 'essential oils' which she then used to poison herself.[101] Despite precautions, patients on trial discharge still killed themselves, such as two Ticehurst patients; one threw himself into the sea, the other out of a window.[102] David S., a married agricultural labourer from Worplesdon, Surrey, was admitted to Brookwood on 1 June 1876, diagnosed as suffering from mania with GPI. He was deemed to be suicidal. After three weeks he tried to escape but by September he was reportedly settled, quiet, rational and working around the asylum. This apparent improvement allowed him to be conditionally discharged on the 16 February 1877 on one month's probation. He was then officially discharged as 'recovered' only to commit suicide by drowning on 28 March. The verdict of the enquiry was 'Suicide while of unsound mind'.[103] A 29-year-old curate, Richard H., was admitted to Holloway Sanatorium suffering from acute mania. He was allegedly violent to others but not to himself, despite refusing food and needing to be fed by tube. Treatments included sulphonal, whisky and electric therapy during his twelve-month stay. He was discharged recovered but elected to stay on as a boarder for a short time before he resumed his career in Holy Orders. In October 1903, the *Daily Mail* reported that he had hanged himself with his stole, observing that the year before, a 'love trouble' had precipitated an earlier unsuccessful suicide attempt by poisoning.[104]

Conclusion

During the course of the nineteenth century, suicidal inclinations and insanity became closely linked in the minds of medical men and, arguably, those of the lay public. Between one-quarter and one-third of all admissions to pauper asylums were listed as 'suicidal' even though 'dangerousness' (either to self or others) was not a criterion required by English law for confinement. During the mid-Victorian period, families, police, clergy and local medical practitioners acted individually, or in concert, to confine individuals as a preventive measure in response to acts of self-violence or threats to do so. Success is difficult to measure, and more work is required on the prevalence of suicide amongst discharged patients, who had previously been described as suicidal whilst incarcerated. The apparent lack of desire for suicide or self-harm was clearly a determinant in the superintendent's decision to release patients, yet as we have seen, some patients succumbed to this impulse once they were released.

Brookwood Asylum patients, in particular, were labelled 'suicidal' for a variety of reasons. Such categorization may have been strategically employed by Poor Law officials to manipulate the rules of the confinement process, as workhouses, too, struggled with overcrowding and were able to deal with only the most quiescent lunatics. The research supports the view, advanced by Olive Anderson, that asylums provided secure locations of surveillance and control of suicidal individuals, women and men who had either attempted suicide, or had threatened to do so. As the non-restraint movement and moral treatment became entrenched in public asylums by mid-century, asylum staff adopted a range of strategic measures to prevent suicides within the institutions, which were increasingly sought as a temporary place of refuge for those disordered in mind.

The evidence, from Brookwood especially, shows that although many patients were allegedly self-destructive, actual suicides within the walls of the asylum were comparatively rare and official statistics confirmed that suicide rates in asylums declined sharply between 1867 and 1911.[105] Earlier in the century, restraint had been commonly used, but with its demise, medical superintendents were obliged to employ other means to prevent suicides within their institutions. During the period under question, strict surveillance was crucial and this was increasingly combined with the use of sedatives and other interventions.[106]

Dealing with suicidal tendencies was usually the responsibility of medical practitioners within the prison and asylum systems, all of whom approached the problem with different clinical criteria.[107] Once identified as suicidal, the nineteenth-century medical profession increasingly saw institutionalized care, with the benefits of specialized diet, regular exercise and removal from the familiar environmental causes, as the correct course of action for these patients. Although there was broad consensus that 'careful watching' of suicidally inclined patients was pivotal, the debate continued as to whether all those who were suicidal were also of unsound mind. Westcott concluded, somewhat sarcastically, 'It may only be a coincidence, but it is a fact, that almost without exception the supporters of the theory that all suicides are insane have been medical attendants in asylums'.[108]

This comparative study of suicide and suicide management at Brookwood and Holloway has again highlighted differences between the two institutions. Before arriving at Brookwood, the workhouse was often the first port of call for poorer families seeking institutional care and control of suicidal relatives. At Holloway, families were more likely to deal directly with the medical profession, although in the first instance this may have taken the form of single care.[109] The inclusion of letters and testimonials in some patient case notes indicates that evidence of suicidal propensity provided by the patients' families was not always trusted. Occasionally, evidence was clearly discounted and not included in the original certificates; this came to light at the inquest into the suicide of Eliza S., one of the ill-fated double suicides at Holloway Sanatorium.

The causes assigned by medical men to explain suicidal tendency differed for the sexes; for men 'the vices, money trouble' and for women 'the passions, remorse, and shame', all of which were associated with the evils of city dwelling and its glamorous but dangerous lure for the morally inept.[110] Anderson refuted the importance of any significant distinction of suicide rates between urban and rural locations, but in the nineteenth century Westcott felt justified in concluding that there was 'one-third more suicide in London than the country', and certainly most patients in these two asylums originated from the towns.[111] The evidence from the admissions records of Brookwood show that the majority of patients admitted between 1867 and 1881 came from the south London workhouses, so that the term 'suicidal', which was widely used, must be viewed with a degree of contextual sensitivity. Such terminology, along with the phrase 'dangerous to others' was used to endorse workhouse authorities' decisions to transfer difficult patients to the (more costly) county asylum. Many workhouses were neither equipped nor willing to deal with the most violent and suicidal insane inmates; nearly all of those who were transferred from the metropolitan workhouses to Brookwood were described as maniacal and suicidal. Once incarcerated, however, many of the same suicidal patients failed to exhibit these tendencies, and the extra precautions so often recommended in contemporary medical publications remained unimplemented. Punitive measures were taken on occasion, and the impression is that drug therapy was increasingly used to impose order and control within the asylum.

It is clear that the term 'suicidal' on the admission orders of patients included a wide range of behaviours and associated risks, described as 'doubtful' by Brushfield in 1879. Many Victorian commentators believed that the 'true' rate of suicidality was closer to 5 per cent. The evidence from these two particular institutions may also suggest a class dynamic in the ascription of suicidal behaviour and the element of risk. In the ongoing negotiation between workhouse and asylum authorities (who both had to deal with institutional overcrowding), it is plausible that workhouse authorities may have exaggerated the danger of suicide in order to secure a bed. There appears to have been a lower rate of 'suicidal' admissions to private asylums. Fewer new patients were initially described as suicidal at Holloway Sanatorium, but over a third suffered from melancholia, which was strongly associated with self-destruction. Constant surveillance was widely considered to be the only effective method to prevent suicide, yet Rees Philipps refused to fully implement this strategy which he viewed as intrusive for his middle-class patients, as well as ineffective. Given the origins of the Holloway patients, Rees Philipps was particularly conscious of such sensitivities. Further, he believed that surveillance could actually stimulate a patient's suicidal propensity. When suicidal behaviour was observed and recorded, it was usually seen at the justification for a series of precautions; a suicide caution would be issued and a companion or attendant slept in the suicidal patient's room. Underlining this, however, was the medical staff's acute awareness of the social status of their patients, so that the weapon of surveillance in the battle against institutional suicide was employed reluctantly. Within a relatively short period of time and in spite of the high staff-to-patient ratios, this relative freedom led to more opportunities for determined patients, so that several notable fatalities and 'accidents' occurred that were considered 'unavoidable' by the superintendent.

CONCLUSION

Located within a short distance of each other, Holloway Sanatorium's grandeur was in stark contrast to the relative plainness and functionality of Brookwood Asylum. The two Surrey asylums coped in distinctive ways with the pressures exerted by patients, families and central administrative authorities. Brookwood was accountable to ratepayers, and its treatment regime was subject to approval by the Commissioners in Lunacy, the Metropolitan Asylum Board (MAB), and the individual Poor Law unions. Holloway offered facilities that might have been enjoyed by the middle class at a country hotel or Continental health resort. Both institutions immediately proved to be more popular than had been expected, which brought the threat of overcrowding. The disruption and inconvenience of the ensuing building work, which went on for lengthy periods of time, militated against the development of stable treatment regimes. It was almost impossible for the superintendents to keep treatment at the forefront, while they oversaw the construction work (which entailed measures to keep patients safe from injury), and, for Brookwood at least, the ever-burgeoning paperwork that a centralized asylum system demanded.

More patients meant more staff, and considerable care was taken by both asylums to recruit reliable and efficient men and women with the right personal qualities. The point of treatment at these two contrasting institutions was broadly the same. They might have cared for vastly different numbers and classes of patients, but both tried to return their patients to whatever constituted normality for them, be it a meagre existence in Bermondsey, or a comfortable life in Walton-on-Thames. To this end, the quality of the staff recruited, trained and retained, was of the first importance, and both managements strove to engage the best attendants and nurses that resources would permit. The care provided by both Brookwood and Holloway was aided by the long service of their first medical superintendents, who provided stability and continuity. The development of staff training is one remarkable aspect of the changing employment opportunities at the asylums. Qualifications brought advantages to the attendants, both financially and in terms of occupational mobility and opportunity. Women, in particular, could enjoy a level of job security and independence that was notably lacking in other areas of employment that were open to them in the nineteenth century. Asylums were one of the few places (outside the small family business, farm or the large stately home), where married couples could work together in the same environment. This potential for secure, 'family' treatment, in turn, brought benefits to groups of patients who were cared for in cottage-style accommodation within the asylum grounds.

Management scrutinized all aspects of the attendants' lives and behaviour. This high level of control, combined with the isolated nature of asylum life, induced the potential for long-serving staff members to become almost as institutionalized as their charges. Staff discipline was, in general, strict at Brookwood and Holloway, and dismissal for misconduct was not unusual. However, the unique strains inherent in caring for the mentally ill did prompt compassion and understanding on the part of the authorities, and these tensions may explain the identifiable inconsistencies in treatment of those staff who transgressed. The anomalies might also be explained by the fact that – once trained – a skilled attendant had better prospects in the external job market. Keeping trained staff was a constant battle, and leeway was given to the good worker, as suggested by the apparent leniency with which some offences were dealt.

In its engagement of genteel companions, Holloway had one group of staff that would not have been contemplated at Brookwood. Prized not for their professional skills, but rather for their social status and shared middle-class values and habits, these companions represent a unique stratum within the asylum hierarchy. Their appointment was ostensibly therapeutic in that it was hoped that their example would encourage the patients to return to middle-class normality. It was also intended to make life pleasant for the patients, as well as offer employment to distressed gentlefolk, and had implications for the level of supervision at Holloway. The sanatorium offered discrete, almost unobtrusive care, partially due to the high staffing levels, and the companions were engaged as informal escorts rather than custodians. Brookwood's restricted complement of staff shaped a regime of care that was more vigilant and regimented than at its neighbour. The middle-class patients at Holloway were offered almost one-to-one care and enjoyed relative freedom, partially as a result of the superintendent's reluctance to employ full surveillance. However, this had an unfortunate impact on their safety. Brookwood certainly had more 'accidents' than Holloway, but the sanatorium's suicide rate was higher.

Brookwood's public accountability, and the unavoidable conservatism of a state-run organization, meant that it was disadvantaged compared to Holloway, with its ability to explore new treatments, develop staff education protocols, and experiment with engaging women doctors and paid companions. Where every appointment was a matter of public scrutiny, the management of Brookwood had to justify any addition to the payroll.

Gender was not the primary determining factor in admissions, treatment and outcome at either Brookwood Asylum or Holloway Sanatorium. The detailed examination of the patient composition at Brookwood and Holloway established that the male and female admissions were roughly equal, reflecting the sex ratio in the general population, and were comparable to other lunatic asylums. Women were *not* disproportionally represented; however, some aspects of incarceration remained unique to each sex. In both institutions, women accounted for a much larger proportion of the patients who remained in the asylum for an extended period. This may have had more to do with the intent of admission than their sex or the nature of their illness. As in metropolitan workhouse infirmaries, significant numbers of males of working age were admitted and generally had been employed before entering the workhouse. Arguably, they were treated with the intention of returning them to useful employment as soon as possible. The working history of female patients (particularly at Brookwood) was rarely documented, and this neglect is mirrored in other Victorian records, most notably in the decennial census returns. If they were not regularly employed, perhaps there was not the same urgency to return them to society. There is a predominance of single and widowed patients, particularly of women in this category, which might indicate that being married could militate against incarceration for women, especially those in middle age.

The nineteenth-century asylum aimed to contain, care for, and ultimately cure its patients. In this, Brookwood and Holloway were typical, and the profile of illness and disease is also typical in both institutions. Brookwood and Holloway admitted patients whose mental illness had the same or similar underlying causes, but Brookwood had a higher ratio of patients whose illness was attributable to poverty and deprivation. Admission from the workhouses meant that many of its patients were in poor physical condition, in addition to being mentally ill, and this compromised the treatment possibilities and outcome. Alcohol was blamed as a contributory factor in more cases at Brookwood than Holloway, which, it might be argued, reflects the centrality of drink in the lifestyle of the poor in the Victorian age.

As with all nineteenth-century organizations, statistics were taken as the reliable measure of effectiveness. Recovery and death rates were rigorously recorded, being perceived to a large extent as indicators of the success of treatment. Brookwood may have been more constrained than Holloway in what it could do, but it strove to the limit of its resources to provide a safe and curative environment. To a large extent the death rates at Brookwood and Holloway were dictated by the class, previous medical history and circumstances of the patients. Many patients – especially men of working age – arrived at Brookwood in a compromised physical state, which no amount of asylum care could remedy. Holloway compared unfavourably with Brookwood in its deferential neglect of would-be suicides, which provided opportunity for those who were determined to end their lives.

The managers of Brookwood went beyond their remit as mere custodians of the insane; it was their intention to run – as far as possible – a curative organization. Both institutions offered aspects of moral therapy encompassing the physical environment, diet, exercise and spiritual guidance. Holloway Sanatorium's patients and their families expected a modern, high-class facility with the most up-to-date treatments and imaginative therapies. The newest drugs were used more widely than at Brookwood, as financial constraints were fewer, although the relative paucity of drug therapies at Brookwood may have reflected the superintendent's own beliefs rather than MAB dictates.

In some respects, the patients' experience at Brookwood reflects that at Buckinghamshire County Asylum, as outlined by David Wright. As Wright has pointed out, asylum incarceration for 40–60 per cent of patients lasted for twelve months or less.[1] Laurence Ray's comparison of pauper patients in Brookwood and Lancaster Asylum noted how the long-term confinement of patients was exceptional.[2] Given these studies, it is remarkable how the image of lengthy incarceration has persisted and how it was exploited by historians to suggest that women, in particular, fell victim to discriminatory practices and were over-represented in asylum admissions.[3] These claims are confounded in this study, which shows that women outnumber men by only a small fraction. Where recovery did not occur soon after admission, however, they were likely to be incarcerated for long periods of time. This pattern means that women did form the bulk of residual patients in both Brookwood and Holloway at the end of each year. The slowness of their recovery, natural longevity and their perceived limited options in the outside world – and not their sex – explains their predominance in both asylums' end-of-year returns.

Women tended to stay longer at Holloway than their male counterparts, which might be attributed to the comfort of the surroundings there. The 'right' class of female patient might secure a place at a reduced rate. For the unmarried or widowed woman, the attraction was clear. Her family was largely relieved of the burden of her care, and Holloway was a pleasant alternative to being accommodated on sufferance by family members. Genteel poverty is evidenced by the sanatorium's involvement with the After-Care Association. Where families had money, there is evidence of a remarkably high number of voluntary admissions, which, themselves, entailed complicated negotiations with regard to supervision.

It was surprising to discover that a small number of children were regularly admitted to Brookwood, despite the management's reservations in dealing with them in an adult institution. The proportion of children housed at Brookwood was larger than that identified by Melling in Devon.[4] They were usually there at their family's request and most, unfortunately, died in the institution. Holloway admitted adolescents, but not young children; asylums were essentially an adult experience, and the treatment given in them was designed to deal with adult conditions.

Pauper patients at Brookwood did not necessarily receive second-class treatment. The contemporary concept of respectability modified the kind of stark differentiation in treatment between the classes that might have been expected, since each asylum housed patients who were deemed 'respectable'. An important conclusion is that the asylums' contrasting therapeutic regimes and committal and discharge processes were less evident than a class-based model might have predicted. The two institutions shared many aims and approaches. Brookwood aspired to be more than merely a custodial institution, as directed by Poor Law legislation. In spite of limited resources and budget, for example, the Brookwood doctors undertook the relatively rare procedure of trepanning *in extremis*. Chemical intervention was only given to violent or suicidal cases, the management preferring the more humane (and certainly cheaper) alternative of seclusion. Perhaps more extraordinary is the willingness of Brookwood's doctors to use electrical therapy. At Holloway, despite the higher staff-to-patient ratio and the wider range of available treatments, any suicidally disposed patients there were more at risk than at the nearby county asylum.

Holloway offered comfort to the middle classes with sufficient diversion to keep patients occupied and amused and its guise as a convalescent home encouraged entertainment as therapy. This was in part expected by the patients' families, but it was also an alternative to the work therapy that was intrinsic in state institutions which was not initially seen as appropriate for the middle- and upper-class inmates.[5] Brookwood had a tightly organized work schedule, and recreational therapy was offered less often than labour. Nevertheless, despite its many advantages over Brookwood, its ambiguous nature permitted some serious incidences of neglect and incompetence that resulted in tragedy.

Would-be suicides were enormously difficult to handle, not least because groups of professionals viewed them slightly differently. To the mid-nineteenth-century physician, asylums offered the advantages of controlled diet, exercise and removal from the immediate contributing causes of their psychiatric condition. There was surprisingly little agreement as to whether all those who were intent on self-destruction were necessarily of unsound mind. If a determined suicide was not mad, what justification was there to incarcerate and treat him or her? In their treatment of the suicidal, Brookwood and Holloway's differences are evident. Brookwood patients were invariably admitted via the workhouse, while the relatives and family doctors of the patients brought their would-be suicides directly to Holloway. The family's letters and testimonials to the asylum's management demonstrate that their direct experience of the patient's suicidal symptoms was a powerful factor in their admission.

If suicide and self-harm were indicators of the failure of a supposed cura-tive institution, then neither Brookwood nor Holloway were wholly successful. The apparent freedom from the impulse to commit suicide clearly influenced decisions on discharge, although this gamble (if such it was), has been seen here to have resulted in some completed suicides of those just released. The research here supports Olive Anderson's view that the security and overview offered by Victorian asylums made them increasingly attractive as temporary refuges for those disordered in mind.[6] The common instance of the label 'suicidal', however, leads one to question whether it was employed by Poor Law officials to get all but the most passive of lunatics out of the workhouse.

The evidence from Brookwood strongly indicates that this might have been the case. While suicidal propensity featured prominently in the admis-sion records, completed suicides within the asylum were comparatively rare. Between 1867 and 1881 many of Brookwood's patients came via south London workhouses and nearly all those transferred were described as dangerous and/ or suicidal. Once in the asylum, they rarely showed any such tendencies, and extra precautions for their safety proved unnecessary. Official statistics confirm that asylum suicide rates declined sharply between 1867 and 1911. It might be argued that this attests to the success of asylums in suicide prevention, or that difficult patients were transferred under the heading 'suicidal' as it was the easiest and most convenient way in which to deal with intractable lunatics. The demise of physical restraint in this period might also have had its part to play; no longer able to tie up the patient, strict surveillance and sedatives made it more diffi-cult for the determined suicide to succeed. However one accepts the correctness truth of the term 'suicidal' on the admission orders of patients, it seems to have covered many types of behaviour.

Suicide rates were also relatively low at Holloway, although this must be tem-pered with the fact that a far smaller percentage of admissions were given the 'suicidal' label. Where the danger was judged significant, extra surveillance was ordered and companions accompanied the patients, day and night. The social status of the patients, and the staff's reluctance to be seen to be heavy handed and disrespectful, interfered with the level and effectiveness of surveillance. The opportunity to self-harm was taken by some patients, and fatalities resulted.

Social class – rather than gender – was the major determinant in terms of patients admitted, and their treatment. This is the core theme and outcome of the book, which demonstrates that the treatment of pauper lunatics and those of 'the middling sort' was provided in a manner considered appropriate for each class. The rigid class distinctions of Victorian daily life were reflected in the two institutions. Such differentiation contributed to the accepted view that it was both appropriate and medically beneficial to ensure that middle-class patients were segregated from insane paupers. However, this distinction was not set in stone, and, in reality, was less rigidly adhered to than theories of segregation by class would suggest.

There were remarkable similarities between the two institutions: the ratio of men and women, the age profile of the patients, and the average length of stay are broadly comparable. Outcomes are also similar, and it is striking that the failure to attain early release generally meant a protracted period in both asylums. The superintendents of Brookwood and Holloway strove, according to the means at their disposal, to provide a curative regime. Neither was interested in the permanent incarceration of their charges, and they were sufficiently well informed with developments in the care of the mentally ill to adapt treatment to take into account current theories and therapies.

The asylum environment, as investigated here, has revealed a nuanced picture of the complexities of nineteenth-century custodial care for the insane. The evidence presented in *Institutionalizing the Insane* goes some way to mitigate the image of the asylum as a harsh, non-curative warehouse, particularly with regard to the pauper Brookwood Asylum. There were difficulties and errors of judgement, but some patients had the opportunity to recuperate from the punitive realities of their external existences. In their respective ways, this was potentially the case for the patients of all classes.

The differences between Brookwood and Holloway are acknowledged in this book but some similarities are highlighted, thereby confounding long-held theories, while reinforcing others. All actors must be considered; the evidence from letters written to and from the patients has provided an important and often-missing perspective. This is especially so with regard to those associated with the Brookwood inmates which have not only revealed the complexities of individual family circumstances, but have also shown the wide-ranging emotions involved. The extent of the families' interaction with asylum authorities as well as the levels of literacy has also challenged assumptions that Brookwood cared only for 'pauper' patients. The written correspondence has provided a rare opportunity to hear patients' voices, which casts a different light on the reality of institutional psychiatric care in the nineteenth century that cannot be provided by administrative records alone. This recognition has stimulated a growing research interest in the patient experience of mental ill-health, and the material from Brookwood Asylum and Holloway Sanatorium that has been used here, has enabled a process of highlighting the critical importance, and interdependence, of medical, official and lay narratives.

NOTES

Introduction: Contexts of Insanity

1. 'Report of the Lancet Commission on Lunatic Asylums: Brookwood Asylum', *Lancet*, 2 (4 December 1875), pp. 816–20, on p. 817.
2. J. Melling, 'Accommodating Madness: New Research in the Social History of Insanity and Institutions', in J. Melling and W. Forsythe (eds), *Insanity, Institutions and Society, 1800–1914: A Social History of Madness in Comparative Perspective* (London and New York: Routledge, 1999), pp. 1–30.
3. M. Foucault, *Madness and Civilisation: A History of Insanity in the Age of Reason*, trans. R. Howard (London: Tavistock, 1965); C. Jones and R. Porter (eds), *Reassessing Foucault: Power, Medicine, and the Body* (London: Routledge, 1994); D. Wright, 'Getting out of the Asylum: Understanding the Confinement of the Insane in the Nineteenth Century', *Social History of Medicine*, 10:1 (1997), pp. 137–55.
4. Melling, 'Accommodating Madness', p. 7.
5. A. T. Scull, *Museums of Madness: The Social Organization of Insanity in Nineteenth-Century England* (London: Allen Lane, 1979).
6. A. T. Scull, *The Most Solitary of Afflictions: Madness and Society in Britain, 1700–1900* (New Haven, CT, and London: Yale University Press, 1993); A. Scull, C. MacKenzie and N. Hervey, *Masters of Bedlam: The Transformation of the Mad-Doctoring Trade* (Princeton, NJ: Princeton University Press, 1996). Foucault argued that this growth resulted from the regulation of the working class by emergent bourgeois intellectuals, a group which Scull saw as including asylum superintendents hungry for professional recognition.
7. J. Melling and W. Forsythe, *The Politics of Madness, the State, Insanity and Society in England, 1845–1914* (London: Routledge, 2006); A. Scull, 'Rethinking the History of Asylumdom', in Melling and Forsythe (eds), *Insanity, Institutions and Society*, pp. 295–315, on pp. 296–9.
8. J. Andrews and A. Digby (eds), *Sex and Seclusion, Class and Custody: Perspectives on Gender and Class in the History of British and Irish Psychiatry* (Amsterdam and New York: Rodopi, 2004). See their introduction for an expansive discussion.
9. L. D. Smith, *'Cure, Comfort and Safe Custody': Public Lunatic Asylums in Early Nineteenth-Century England* (London: Leicester University Press, 1999).
10. P. Bartlett, *The Poor Law of Lunacy: The Administration of Pauper Lunatics in Mid-Nineteenth-Century England* (London: Leicester University Press, 1999).

11. A. Digby, *Madness, Morality and Medicine: A Study of the York Retreat, 1796–1914* (Cambridge: Cambridge University Press, 1985); C. MacKenzie, *Psychiatry for the Rich: A History of Ticehurst Private Asylum, 1792–1917* (London and New York: Routledge, 1992).

12. Scull, *The Most Solitary of Afflictions*, p. 354.

13. L. Walsh, 'A Class Apart? Admissions to the Dundee Royal Lunatic Asylum', in Andrews and Digby (eds), *Sex and Seclusion*, pp. 249–70, on p. 265.

14. Melling and Forsythe, *The Politics of Madness*; P. Michael, 'Class, Gender and Insanity in Nineteenth-Century Wales', in Andrews and Digby (eds), *Sex and Seclusion*, pp. 95–122, on p. 115.

15. Walsh, 'A Class Apart?' p. 265.

16. Andrews and Digby (eds), *Sex and Seclusion*, p. 9.

17. E. Showalter, *The Female Malady: Women, Madness and English Culture, 1830–1980* (London: Virago, 1987); J. Ussher, *Women's Madness: Misogyny or Mental Illness?* (Hemel Hempstead: Harvester Wheatsheaf, 1991).

18. In nineteenth-century British India, for example, Waltraud Ernst has highlighted the importance of contextualizing male and female maladies and relating them to other factors, including class. W. Ernst, 'European Madness and Gender in Nineteenth-Century British India', *Social History of Medicine*, 9:3 (1996), pp. 357–82, on p. 81.

19. J. K. Walton, 'Casting Out and Bringing Back in Victorian England: Pauper Lunatics, 1840–1870', in W. F. Bynum, R. Porter and M. Shepherd (eds), *The Anatomy of Madness: Essays in the History of Psychiatry, Vol. 2, Institutions and Society* (London: Routledge Keegan and Paul, 1985), pp. 132–46.

20. Wright, 'Getting Out of the Asylum', p. 153.

21. E. Dwyer, *Homes for the Mad: Life inside Two Nineteenth-Century Asylums* (New Brunswick, NJ: Rutgers University Press, 1987).

22. Melling and Forsythe, *The Politics of Madness*.

23. G. Mooney and J. Reinarz (eds), *Permeable Walls: Historical Perspectives on Hospital and Asylum Visiting* (Amsterdam and New York: Rodopi, 2009).

24. Anne Digby's study of the York Retreat was the first to computerize all patient records. Digby, *Madness, Morality and Medicine*. Other historians who have followed her lead include David Wright with his work on the Bucks County Asylum, and the research team of Joseph Melling and Bill Forsythe on the Devon County Asylum.

25. There were several missing case books, especially with regard to chronic patients and voluntary boarders so that it was not always possible to follow a case through to its conclusion. Staff registers were only available from 1895 and appear to not have been updated regularly.

26. A. Shepherd, 'Writing the Asylum', work in progress.

27. MacKenzie, *Psychiatry for the Rich*, p. 2.

28. L. Wannell, 'Patients' Relatives and Psychiatric Doctors: Letter Writing in the York Retreat, 1875–1910', *Social History of Medicine*, 20:2 (2007), pp. 297–313, on p. 299.

29. This is followed by more detailed data and analysis in Chapters 3 and 4.

30. E. Renvoize, 'The Association of Medical Officers of Asylums and Hospitals for the Insane, the Medico-Psychological Association and their Presidents', in G. E. Berrios and H. Freeman (eds), *150 Years of British Psychiatry 1841–1991* (London: Tavistock, 1991), pp. 29–78, on p. 69.

31. S. York, 'Alienists, Attendants and the Containment of Suicide in Public Lunatic Asylums, 1845–1890', *Social History of Medicine*, 25:2 (2012), pp. 324–42.

32. D. Wright, *Mental Disability in Victorian England: The Earlswood Asylum, 1847–1901* (Oxford: Oxford University Press, 2001), p. 100.

33. Wright, 'Getting Out of the Asylum'.

34. Parry-Jones observed that over one thousand children and adolescents were admitted to Bethlem from 1815 to 1899. W. L. Parry-Jones, 'The History of Child and Adolescent Psychiatry: Its Present Day Relevance', *Journal of Child Psychology and Psychiatry*, 30:1 (1989), pp. 3–11.

35. L. J. Ray, 'Models of Madness in Victorian Asylum Practice', *European Journal of Sociology*, 22 (1981), pp. 229–64, on p. 234. Wright, 'Getting Out of the Asylum', pp. 143–4.

36. C. MacKenzie, 'Social Factors in the Admission, Discharge, and Continuing Stay of Patients at Ticehurst Asylum, 1845–1917', in F. W. Bynum, R. Porter and M. Shepherd, *The Anatomy of Madness, Vol. 2, Institutions and Society* (London: Tavistock, 1985), pp. 147–74, on p. 159.

37. Walsh, 'A Class Apart?'. Walsh's research shows the ambiguities of class by highlighting the importance of respectability and social propriety as determinants in patient selection.

38. Andrews and Digby (eds), *Sex and Seclusion*, p. 9.

39. See H. Marland, *Dangerous Motherhood: Insanity and Childbirth in Victorian Britain* (Basingstoke and New York: Palgrave Macmillan, 2004).

40. This symptom of anorexia appears in R. Dunglison, *A Dictionary of Medical Sciences* (Philadelphia, PA: Blanchard and Lea, 1856), J. J. Brumberg, *Fasting Girls: The Emergence of Anorexia Nervosa as a Modern Disease* (London: Harvard University Press, 1988), p. 101. Its emergence as a 'modern disease' in the 1870s is attributed to William Gull, although subsequently there has been some debate as to whether it is Gull or the French neuropsychiatrist Ernest Charles Lasègue who deserves to be credited with this discovery. Although the contributions of both show a remarkable but independent coincidence around 1873, Gull is usually associated with the disease based on a rather vague mention of a condition similar to anorexia in a paper read in 1868. W. Vandereycken and R. van Deth, 'Who Was the First to Describe Anorexia Nervosa: Gull or Lasègue?' *Psychological Medicine*, 19:4 (November 1989), pp. 837–45.

41. D. MacKinnon, '"Amusements are Provided": Asylum Entertainment and Recreation in Australia and New Zealand, c. 1860–c. 1945', in Mooney and Reinarz (eds), *Permeable Walls*, pp. 267–88.

42. A. Shepherd and D. Wright, 'Madness, Suicide and the Victorian Asylum: Attempted Self-Murder in the Age of Non-Restraint', *Medical History*, 46:2 (April 2002), pp. 175–96.

43. O. Anderson, *Suicide in Victorian and Edwardian England* (Oxford: Clarendon Press, 1987), esp. ch. 11.

44. Ibid.

45. Shepherd and Wright, 'Madness, Suicide and the Victorian Asylum'; York, 'Alienists, Attendants and the Containment of Suicide'; J. Weaver and D. Wright (eds), *Histories of Suicide: International Perspectives on Self-Destruction in the Modern World* (Toronto: University of Toronto Press, 2009).

46. J. Andrews, 'Case Notes, Case Histories, and Patients' Experience of Insanity at Gartnavel Royal Asylum, Glasgow, in the Nineteenth Century', *Social History of Medicine*, 11 (1998), pp. 255–81, on p. 280.

47. See P. Bartlett, 'The Asylum, the Workhouse and the Voices of the Insane Poor in Nineteenth-Century England', *International Journal of Law and Psychiatry*, 21 (1998), pp. 421–32; C. Coleborne, 'Families, Patients and Emotions: Asylums for the Insane

in Colonial Australia and New Zealand, c. 1880–1910', Social History of Medicine, 19 (2006), pp. 425–42; D. Hirst and P. Michael, 'Family, Community and the Lunatic in Mid-Nineteenth-Century North Wales', in P. Bartlett and D. Wright (eds), Outside the Walls of the Asylum: The History of Care in the Community 1750–2000 (London: Athlone, 1999), pp. 66–85; C. Smith, 'Family, Community and the Victorian Asylum: A Case Study of the Northampton General Lunatic Asylum and its Pauper Lunatics', Family and Community History, 9:2 (2006), pp. 109–24; L. D. Smith, '"Your Very Thankful Inmate": Discovering the Patients of an Early County Lunatic Asylum', Social History of Medicine, advanced access, 3 June 2008, at http://shm.oxfordjournals.org/cgi/content/full/hkn030v1 [accessed 9 July 2008]; Wannell, 'Patients' Relatives and Psychiatric Doctors'.

1 Caring for Surrey's Insane: Brookwood Asylum and Holloway Sanatorium

1. This was also referred to as Wandsworth Asylum and latterly Springfield by c. 1918. I. Lodge Patch, 'The Surrey County Lunatic Asylum (Springfield): Early Years in the Development of an Institution', British Journal of Psychiatry, 159 (1991), 159, pp. 69–77, on p. 70.
2. G. M. Ayers, England's First State Hospitals and the Metropolitan Asylums Board, 1867–1930 (London: Wellcome Institute of the History of Medicine, 1971).
3. J. Taylor, Building for Healthcare: Hospital and Asylum Architecture in England 1840–1914 (London and New York: Mansell, 1991), p. 35.
4. Ibid.
5. Scull, The Most Solitary of Afflictions.
6. Figures taken from the 1801 and 1901 Census Returns.
7. In 1889, authority for Brookwood passed from Surrey Quarter Sessions to the new Surrey County Council.
8. Information compiled from various editions of Gazetteer of England and Wales, available online at www.visionofbritain.org.uk.
9. See H. J. Dyos, Victorian Suburb: A Study of the Growth of Camberwell (Leicester: Leicester University Press, 1961).
10. Anon., 'Visiting Physicians to County Asylums', Asylum Journal, 1 (1854), p. 36; C. Philo, '"Fit Localities for an Asylum": The Historical Geography of the Nineteenth-Century "Mad-Business" in England as Viewed through the Pages of the Asylum Journal', Journal of Historical Geography, 13:4 (1987), pp. 398–415.
11. First Annual Report of Brookwood Asylum for 1867, Wellcome Library for the History of Medicine, [hereafter WLM] WLM28 BE5 S96, pp. 10–11.
12. Ibid.
13. Committee of Justices, 1859, quoted in Patch, 'The Surrey County Lunatic Asylum (Springfield)', p. 71.
14. Ibid.
15. Brookwood Asylum, Report of the Workhouse Accommodation Committee to the Guildford Board of Guardians 1860, Surrey History Centre (SHC) Acc. 6277/70, pp. 6–7.
16. Ibid., p. 11.

17. Brookwood Asylum, Surrey Quarter Session: Minutes of Committee of Visitors of Brookwood Asylum, 1867–1893, 30 May 1867, SHC Acc. 1523/1/9/1–6, p. 12. C. H. Howell, Brookwood's architect and Surrey County Surveyor, also had to ensure that the accommodation was of an adequate standard and size. National Archives, MH83/260.

18. The London Necropolis and Mausoleum Company owned Brookwood Cemetery, a 2,000 acre site that, from 1852, was designed to relieve London's overcrowded church-yards. One of its most distinguishing features was the Brookwood Cemetery Railway that ran from Waterloo Station and was operational from 1854 until the mid-1940s.

19. Charles Henry Howell (1823–1905), County Surveyor for Surrey, FRIBA, also designed Kingston County Hall in 1893, and Surrey's third county asylum, Cane Hill, in 1883–4.

20. Brookwood Annual Report 1867, p. 7.

21. This is examined in detail in Chapter 4.

22. W. L. Parry-Jones, *The Trade in Lunacy: A Study of Private Madhouses in England in the Eighteenth and Nineteenth Centuries* (London: Routledge and Kegan Paul, 1972).

23. C. N. French, *The Story of St Luke's Hospital* (London: W. Heinemann, 1951), p. 8.

24. S. Low, *The Charities of London* (London: Sampson Low, Son, and Marston, 1867), p. 33.

25. Digby, *Madness, Morality and Medicine*.

26. Anthony Ashley Cooper, seventh Earl of Shaftesbury, KG (1801–85) was concerned with the welfare of the insane for a period of over sixty years, an important period for the development of relevant legislation. He first became involved with the cause in 1827 as a member of a select committee reviewing the condition of pauper lunatics. He was appointed one of the fifteen newly created Metropolitan Commissioners, later going on to become the first chairman of the Commissioners in Lunacy, a post he held for the remainder of his life. See *ODNB*.

27. *Surrey Advertiser*, 20 June 1885, SHC Acc. 6277/4/0.

28. J. Elliot, *Palaces, Patronage and Pills – Thomas Holloway: His Sanatorium, College and Picture Gallery* (Egham: Royal Holloway, 1996).

29. Ibid.

30. Ibid., p. 8.

31. A. Harrison-Barbet, *Thomas Holloway, Victorian Philanthropist* (Egham: Royal Hollo-way, 1994), p. 80.

32. A. Saint, 'Holloway Sanatorium: A Conservation Nightmare', *Victorian Society Annual* (1993), pp. 19–34. James Beal was instrumental in the campaign for governmental reforms in 1870s and acted as Holloway's public relations agent in matters concerning both the College and the Sanatorium.

33. Elliot, *Palaces, Patronage and Pills*, p. 23.

34. Shaftesbury was chairman of the Commissioners in Lunacy from 1845 to 1885.

35. Under his editorship (1844–83), George Godwin transformed the *Builder* into the most successful specialist paper of its kind, with an extensive and varied readership. Arti-cles focused on new buildings, architectural debates, archaeology, history and the arts. The *Builder* was also well known for its campaigns for health and housing, supporting schemes such as charitable trust housing, public baths and pavilion-plan hospitals. Both in the journal and in articles published elsewhere, Godwin, like Holloway, frequently endorsed his belief in individual endeavour and perseverance.

36. 'How to Spend a Quarter of a Million, or More', *Builder* (25 March 1871), xxix, 1468, p. 220; 'How Best to Spend Money for the Public Good?', *Builder* (15 April 1871), xxix,

1471, pp. 277–9, on p. 277; 'In What Way Can Good Best be Done?', *Builder* (22 April 1871), xxix, 1472, pp. 297–8, on p. 297.

37. *Builder* (15 April 1871), xxix, 1471, pp. 277–9, on p. 277.

38. 'Suggestions and Instructions in Reference to a Proposed Lunatic Asylum at St Ann's Heath, near Virginia Water Station, Surrey', Holloway papers, 1872, SHC Acc. 2620/6/1, p. 15.

39. For example he was concerned as to the effectiveness of the drying and airing closets and advised that the best were to be found at Bridgend Asylum, suggesting that competition entrants should view them accordingly. See 'Suggestions and Instructions', SHC Acc. 2620.

40. Ibid., p. 16.

41. William Crossland's architectural practice was centred on Huddersfield, Halifax and Leeds and was responsible for at least fifty-eight designs. These included several ecclesiastical projects, commercial buildings in Huddersfield including the Kirkdale Buildings, two mansions and, perhaps most famously, Rochdale Town Hall, which with its mixture of French, Flemish and English style, served as a precursor for the Sanatorium. The largely obscure architect, John Philpott Jones, by Crossland's own admission contributed significantly to the winning design, having been consulted by Crossland, who had not wanted to enter the competition alone. Jones provided the basic planning while Crossland did the sketch elevations. The London partner of Edward Salmons of Manchester, Jones was involved in the early days of the Sanatorium's construction but he died suddenly in 1874.

42. *Building News and Engineering Journal*, 23:916 (26 July 1872), p. 68.

43. Saint, 'Holloway Sanatorium', p. 21.

44. 'The Competition Designs for Proposed Lunatic Asylums at S. Ann's Heath', *Building News and Engineering Journal*, 23:916 (2 August 1872), pp. 75–7, on p. 75.

45. 'Lunatic Asylum, S. Ann's Heath', *Building News and Engineering Journal*, 23:927 (11 October 1872), p. 282.

46. 'The Holloway Sanatorium, Virginia Water', *Builder*, 25:1797 (14 July 1877), p. 710.

47. Royal Holloway College opened in 1887.

48. J. Taylor, 'The Architect and the Pauper Asylum in Late Nineteenth Century England. G. T. Hine's 1901 Review of Asylum Space and Planning', in L. Topp, J. E. Moran and J. Andrews, *Madness, Architecture and the Built Environment: Psychiatric Spaces in Historical Context* (London: Routledge, 2007), pp. 263–84.

49. Miscellaneous notes, anonymous, SHC Acc. 2620.

50. Formerly Superintendent of Wonford House Hospital, Exeter.

51. By 1884, approximately £900,000 of Holloway's personal fortune had been utilized by his last two projects, £200,000–£300,000 of this spent on the Sanatorium. A widower since 1875, his estate was left to his sister-in-law, Mary Ann Driver, who subsequently transferred it to Henry Driver and George Martin, together with £20,000 for continuation of the business. Both brothers-in-laws had been instrumental in the running of the Holloway business since *c.* 1868 and in 1884 adopted the additional surname of Holloway by deed poll. Harrison-Barbet, *Thomas Holloway*.

52. Smith, *'Cure, Comfort and Safe Custody'*, p. 6.

53. Ibid., p. 7.

54. The Lunacy Act 1845 (8 & 9 Vict., c. 100) and the County Asylums Act 1845.

55. Philo, 'Fit Localities for an Asylum', p. 409.

56. Ibid., p. 404.

57. Ibid., p. 405.
58. Ibid., pp. 410–1.
59. R. Rawlinson, 'Report on the Proposed Site of Surrey Asylum', 13 May 1861, National Archives, MH38/260.
60. Smith, *'Cure, Comfort and Safe Custody'*, p. 33.
61. C. H. Howell, 'Report on the Surrey Asylum', 16 March 1868, National Archives, MH83/260.
62. Brookwood Annual Report 1867, p. 32.
63. Howell, 'Report on the Surrey Asylum', MH83/260.
64. Ibid. This figure was given as being exclusive of fittings, engineers and gas works.
65. Brookwood Annual Report 1867.
66. J. Conolly (series), 'Lectures on the Construction and Government of Lunatic Asylums', reprinted in the *Lancet*, 113 (4 July 1846), pp. 2–5, on p. 2.
67. S. Rutherford, 'Landscapers for the Mind: English Asylum Designers, 1845–1914', *Gardening History*, 33:1 (Summer 2005), pp. 2–19, on p. 2.
68. Brookwood Annual Report 1867, p. 38.
69. Lloyd was virtually unknown outside of asylum design and gardening; his other projects included asylums at Chichester, Middlesbrough, Hill End Hertfordshire and Rauceby in Lincolnshire. Rutherford, 'Landscapers for the Mind', pp. 15–19.
70. See Chapter 2 for more details on Lloyd in this capacity.
71. Brookwood Annual Report 1867, p. 32.
72. *Surrey Advertiser*, 1 April 1875, SHC Acc. 6277/40.
73. Ibid. The hospital had two dormitories with twelve beds, in addition to four single rooms, attendant's accommodation, a scullery, kitchen, etc.
74. Elliot, *Palaces Patronage and Pills*, p. 23.
75. Although no specific place of worship was provided for the relatively smaller number of Roman Catholic patients (most patients were recorded on admission as being 'Church of England'), arrangements were made for the local parish priest to visit the sanatorium on a regular basis.
76. Annual Reports 1886–1906, Minutes of the Annual and Ordinary Meetings of the General Committee for Holloway Sanatorium, SHC Acc. 2620/1/1, 1887, p. 5.
77. 'The Competition Designs for Proposed Lunatic Asylums', p. 75.
78. Holloway Annual Report 1887, SHC Acc. 2620/1/1, p. 5.
79. *Surrey Advertiser*, 20 June 1885, SHC Acc. 6277/4/0.
80. Ibid.
81. John Thompson of Peterborough worked on Holloway College at Mount Lee under Crossland. The chapel is built from the same pink bricks as the college.
82. *Surrey Advertiser*, 20 June 1885, SHC Acc. 6277/4/0.
83. J. Noorthouck, *History of London* (1773), quoted in French, *The Story of St Luke's Hospital*, p. 11. By 1882 the Sanatorium's building costs already reached £300,000 (originally estimated at £40,000); by way of contrast, the private Cotton Hill Asylum, built in 1854, had cost £29,000.
84. 'Holloway College and Sanatorium Virginia Water', *Building News*, 45 (16 September 1881), pp. 393, 356.
85. 'The Holloway Sanatorium', *Builder*, 43:2031 (7 January 1882), pp. 23–4.
86. Ashbee Journals, quoted in Saint, 'Holloway Sanatorium', p. 25. Charles Robert Ashbee (1863–1942) notably founded the Guild of Handicrafts in 1888, and established a com-

mittee for the survey of the memorials of Greater London to guard against the loss of London's historic buildings. This work was continued through the Survey of London.

87. Smith, 'Cure, Comfort and Safe Custody', p. 53.
88. Ibid., pp. 53–4.
89. Ibid., p. 74.
90. Brookwood Asylum, Minutes of Committee of Visitors, SHC Acc. 1523/1/9/1.
91. D. Wright, 'The Certification of Insanity in Nineteenth-Century England and Wales', *History of Psychiatry*, 9 (1998), pp. 267–90, esp. pp. 271–7.
92. Bartlett, *The Poor Law of Lunacy*, p. 41.
93. For more detailed analysis, see Chapters 3 and 4.
94. Brookwood Annual Report 1867, p. 38.
95. Ibid., p. 34.
96. Local Government Act 1888.
97. The findings revealed by the data are discussed in more detail in Chapter 3.
98. F. Driver, *Power and Pauperism: The Workhouse System 1834–1884* (Cambridge: Cambridge University Press, 1993), p. 106.
99. Bartlett, *The Poor Law of Lunacy*, p. 3; W. Forsythe, J. Melling and R. Adair, 'The New Poor Law and the County Pauper Lunatic Asylum: The Devon Experience 1834–1884', *Social History of Medicine*, 9:3 (December 1996), pp. 335–55.
100. Brookwood Annual Report 1869, SHC Acc. 1523/1/1/2/1, p. 9.
101. Brookwood Asylym, Case Books, Females, 1867–1896, SHC Acc. 1523/3/21/1–16 [hereafter Brookwood Female Case Book followed by reference], SHC Acc. 1523/2/21; Brookwood Annual Report 1867.
102. Brookwood Female Case Book, SHC Acc. 1523/3/21/2.
103. Brookwood Annual Report 1868, SHC Acc. 1523/1/1/1.
104. Regulations for the Holloway Sanatorium Approved by the Secretary of State [hereafter Regulations for the Holloway Sanatorium 1886], SHC Acc. 2620, p. 7.
105. See Chapter 3.
106. Holloway, Rules for the Admission, Visiting and Discharge of Patients 1886, SHC Acc. 2620/6/11.
107. MacKenzie, *Psychiatry for the Rich*, p. 207.
108. 'The Holloway Sanatorium', pp. 23–4.
109. Holloway Annual Reports 1886–1906, SHC Acc. 2620/1/1.
110. See Chapter 3.
111. Holloway Annual Report 1886, SHC Acc. 2620/1/1, p. 9.
112. Holloway Minutes of the General Committee, 15 November 1887, SHC Acc. 2620/1/1.
113. The surviving minutes of the General Committee only provide details of patients who were actually admitted, not those who applied and perhaps were refused. Some details are included of those cases where payment arrears occurred, leading to their subsequent removal.
114. Holloway, Copy of the Hospital Rules for the Admission and Visiting of Patients, contained in the Holloway Annual Report 1888, WLM28 BE5H74, p. 50.
115. Wright, 'Getting Out of the Asylum'.
116. Walsh, 'A Class Apart?', p. 251.
117. G. Best, *Mid-Victorian Britain 1851–75* (London: Weidenfeld and Nicholson, 1979), pp. 279–81.
118. Melling, 'Sex and Sensibility'.
119. See Chapter 3 for more detailed information.

120. 'The Holloway Sanatorium', pp. 23–4.

121. Ibid.

122. By the nineteenth century, they still admitted a small number of pauper lunatics, but financial assistance was only offered if patients were believed to be curable within twelve months. J. Andrews, A. Briggs, R. Porter, P. Tucker and K. Waddington, *The History of Bethlem* (London: Routledge,1997), p. 454. Soon after opening, St Luke's was readmitting incurable or uncured patients at a slightly higher weekly charge. French, *The History of St Luke's Hospital*, p. 16.

123. Holloway Sanatorium, Female Case Books, 1885–1910, SHC Acc. 3473/3/1–9 [hereafter Holloway Female Case Book], Eva A., Holloway Female Case Book 1898, SHC Acc. 3473/3/1, 6, 7, p. 29.

124. One study of voluntary patients in France is P. E. Prestwich, 'Family Strategies and Medical Power: "Voluntary" Committal in a Parisian Asylum, 1876–1914,' *Journal of Social History*, 27:4 (June 1994), pp. 797–816.

125. Holloway Female Case Book, Voluntary Boarders, SHC Acc. 3473/3/28.

126. Regulations for the Holloway Sanatorium 1886, SHC Acc. 2620.

127. Rules for the Admission, Visiting and Discharge of Patients 1886, SHC Acc. 2620.

128. Charity Commission Deed, 29 January 1889, SHC Acc. 2620/6/5.

129. Ibid.

130. Holloway Annual Report 1891, SHC Acc. 2620/1/1.

131. Chancery lunatics were those who were of considerable financial means and whose estates were placed under statutory supervision, a procedure which had been utilized since medieval times, although from 1845 they came under the scope of Lunacy Acts.

132. Melling and Forsythe, *The Politics of Madness*, p. 49.

133. P. Michael, *Care and Treatment of the Mentally Ill in North Wales 1800–2000* (Cardiff: University of Wales Press, 2000), pp. 72–3.

134. Most famously, Charles Dickens's account of his visit to St Luke's, recounted in 'A Curious Dance around a Curious Tree', *Household Words* (17 January 1852), pp. 387–8.

135. Brookwood Quarter Session Report 1867, SHC Acc. 1523/1/9/1.

136. Brookwood Annual Report 1887, SHC Acc. 1523/1/1/4, p. 61.The specific reasons why are not made clear.

137. Brookwood Quarter Session Report 1867–68, SHC Acc. 1523/1/9/1.

138. Brookwood Quarter Session Report 1867–68, SHC Acc. 1523/1/9/1.

139. *Surrey Advertiser*, 1 April 1875, SHC Acc. 6277/40.

140. Ibid.

141. Ibid.

142. This is similar to the differentials between Wonford House and the Devon County Asylum, as described by Melling and Forsythe, *The Politics of Madness*, p. 201.

143. Brookwood Report to the Commissioners in Lunacy, 12 December 1867 to August 1 1916, Reports 20 and 21 November 1868, SHC Acc. 1523/1/20, p. 5.

144. Chapter 5 on therapeutics discusses how the financial aspects of foodstuff production created tension with the therapeutic aims of the asylum.

145. J. Walton, *The British Seaside: Holidays and Resorts in the Twentieth Century* (Manchester: Manchester University Press, 2000), p. 29.

146. This became known as St Ann's Hospital, and was designed by Weir Schultz. It opened in 1903 and took up to forty patients. Weir Schultz thereafter was the Sanatorium's architect; in 1903 he oversaw the building of the Male Infirmary, and over the next thirty years he was responsible for many additions and alterations.

147. A small number of female lunatics from the Devon County Asylum stayed in a seaside villa in Exmouth in the summers of 1856 and 1857. Melling and Forsythe, *The Politics of Madness*, p. 53.
148. Holloway Annual Report 1886, SHC Acc. 2620/1/1, p. 10.
149. Holloway Sanatorium, Minutes of the House Committee, 3 January 1887, SHC Acc. 2620/2/1, p. 17.
150. This is discussed in more detail in Chapter 4.
151. MacKenzie, *Psychiatry for the Rich*, p. 141.
152. Papers of George Martin Holloway, Royal Holloway College Archives, GB131/11/1.
153. Holloway Annual Report 1894, SHC Acc. 2620/1/1, p. 100.
154. Although no precise details are available, it is unlikely that numbers rivalled the upper-class Ticehurst Asylum, where, in 1877, twenty-two carriages and thirty-three horses were kept. MacKenzie, *Psychiatry for the Rich*, p. 138.
155. Melling and Forsythe, *The Politics of Madness*.

2 Therapeutic Agents: Doctors and Attendants

1. This originated from the term 'alienation of mind' which can be traced back to the fifteenth century. It remained in medical parlance, albeit less evident, until the 1930s.
2. J. Oppenheim, *'Shattered Nerves': Doctors, Patients and Depression in Victorian England* (Oxford: Oxford University Press, 1991), p. 27.
3. The Medico-Psychological Association finally became the Royal College of Psychiatrists in 1971. Originally the idea of Samuel Hitch, the Association's membership fluctuated over the years; in 1855 there were 121 members but with the opening of many more asylums in the second half of the century, it had increased to 523 by 1894.
4. Its publications commenced in 1853, with the *Asylum Journal*, evolving to the *Asylum Journal of Mental Science*, and then in 1858, the *Journal of Mental Science*. This title was retained until 1963 when it became the *British Journal of Psychiatry*. Oppenheim, *'Shattered Nerves'*, p. 27.
5. Renvoize, 'The Association of Medical Officers', pp. 68–9.
6. Oppenheim, *'Shattered Nerves'*, pp. 25–7.
7. Dwyer, *Homes for the Mad*, p. 83. See also A. Suzuki, *Madness at Home: The Psychiatrist, the Patient and the Family in England, 1820–1860* (Berkeley, CA: University of California Press, 2006).
8. Dwyer, *Homes for the Mad*, p. 83.
9. Elaine Murphy has highlighted the difficulties in the relationship between the Commissioners and local Poor Law officials in her article, which also underlines the financial and practical incentive for workhouse masters. See 'The Lunacy Commissioners and the East London Guardians, 1845–1867, *Medical History*, 46 (2002), pp. 495–524.
10. Brookwood Admissions Registers, SHC Acc. 1523/3/1/1–15. Colney Hatch contained 1,500 patients in 1856; in 1891 Hanwell Asylum had 1,899 patients.
11. A comparison to other private asylums for 1894 showed Holloway to have had the most patients: St Andrew's had 343; Royal Manchester 283; Bethlem 234; St Luke's 191; and Barnwood House 158. Holloway Annual Report 1894, SHC Acc. 2620/1/1.
12. 'Obituary: Thomas Brushfield', *Lancet* (31 December 1910), p. 2054.
13. His initial salary of £600 p.a. rose to £1,000 by 1880. He and his family lived in a large house in the grounds, with all amenities, plus produce from the asylum's farm and gardens, provided.

14. Brushfield was credited with introducing innovative moral treatment at Brookwood that included a strong emphasis on entertainment and activities. His articles included 'On Medical Certificates of Insanity', *Lancet*, 115: 2958 (8 May 1880), pp. 711–3; and 'Practical Hints on the Treatment, Symptoms, and Medico-legal Aspects of Insanity', read before the Chester Medical Society in 1890.

15. G. H. Savage, 'Obituary: Thomas Brushfield', *British Medical Journal* (31 December 1910), p. 2054.

16. Brushfield's son, Thomas Brushfield (1858–1937) also worked in mental health, specializing in mental deficiency. He is accredited for discovering and naming 'Brushfield spots' in children. He was medical superintendent of the Fountain Hospital for Imbeciles, Tooting, from 1914 to 1927.

17. Principles of moral treatment and their implementation at Brookwood and Holloway are discussed further in Chapter 5.

18. A. Digby, 'Moral Treatment at the Retreat, 1796–1846', in W. F. Bynum, R. Porter and M. Shepherd (eds), *The Anatomy of Madness: Essays in the History of Psychiatry: Volume 2: Institutions and Society* (London: Routledge Kegan & Paul, 1985), pp. 52–72, on p. 53.

19. Ray, 'Models of Madness', p. 238.

20. J. M. Granville, *The Care and Cure of the Insane*, 2 vols (London: Hardwicke and Bogue, 1877), vol. 1, p. 58.

21. See Scull, *Museums of Madness*.

22. His salary never exceeded that of his predecessor. Brookwood Register of Officers and Attendants, SHC Acc. 1523/2/2/1, p. 1.

23. Scull, MacKenzie and Hervey, *Masters of Bedlam*, p. 270.

24. Anon., 'Obituary: The Late Sir James M. Moody', *British Journal of Psychiatry* (September 1915), p. 519. He was knighted in 1909 'in recognition of the great advance which he initiated in the care and treatment of the insane'.

25. He retired in 1899 after being obliged to take a year's extended leave due to ill-health.

26. See *British Medical Journal* (23 January 1926), p. 172 for Rees Philipp's obituary.

27. The difficulties surrounding this practice came under very public scrutiny in 1895 with the death of a young male patient. See the case of Thomas W., p. 134, for full details.

28. This can be demonstrated by his views on surveillance and suicidal patients, with occasionally disastrous results.

29. Anon, 'An Asylum and an Elysium', *Woman* (31 August 1892).

30. For example: 1888 opened with 149 patients and 20 boarders. There were 108 admissions that year (58 male, 50 female), plus 85 boarders (50 male, 35 female); 362 patients in total were treated that year. Compared to 1 January 1886, there were 70 patients and boarders resident (30 males and 40 females) but the records are unclear regarding the proportion of certified and voluntary patients for that year. During 1886, 89 patients (37 male, 52 female) and 17 boarders (9 male, 8 female) were admitted. These figures are extrapolated from the Annual Reports and a more extensive analysis of admissions is provided in Chapter 3.

31. Dixon's predecessor was Mr E. F. Cooper, formerly Assistant Medical Officer, St Andrews Hospital, Northampton, a hospital held in high regard by Rees Philipps.

32. Little, previously Assistant MO of Worcester County Asylum was one of forty-eight applicants; Caldecott, previously Resident MO of Eastern Counties Asylum at Colchester, was selected from forty candidates.

33. Holloway Annual Report 1894, SHC Acc. 2620/1/1, p. 103.

34. In return for his services, he received an annual salary of £450, plus lodgings and board; his annual retirement pension was £1,000.
35. Digby, *Madness, Morality and Medicine*, p. 121.
36. Ibid., p. 122.
37. *St Ann's Occasional Magazine*, 33 (Christmas 1896), Holloway Miscellaneous Papers, SHC Acc. 2620/6/23.
38. C. MacKenzie, 'The Life of a Human Football: Women and Madness in the Era of the New Woman', *Society for the Social History of Medicine Bulletin* (1985), pp. 37–40, on p. 37.
39. *Medical Directory 1900*: Jane Buchanan Henderson registered in August 1890, having received her training in London, and Paris (where she had attended Charcot's lectures). Following her three years at Holloway, she worked as Clinical Assistant at the London Throat and Ear Hospital and in outpatients at the New Hospital for Women.
40. Holloway Superintendent's Annual Report 1890, read at the Annual Meeting of the General Committee, 16 February 1891, SHC, open shelves.
41. Emily Louisa Dove began her training at the London School of Medicine for Women in the winter session of 1886, and qualified MB London in 1890. She too worked at the New Hospital for Women, as Resident Medical Officer, and in her later years, appeared to have developed an interest in public health matters, publishing articles on contaminated food and the use of arsenic in wallpaper and textiles.
42. Tasmanian-born Rosina Clara Despard commenced at the London School of Medicine for Women in the summer session of 1891, aged 28. There are no further details of her career as a doctor after 1909.
43. Brookwood Annual Report 1895, SHC Acc. 2620/1/1, p. 113.
44. Ibid.
45. See Chapter 5 for a more detailed consideration of therapeutics.
46. Despite their pivotal role, there has been insufficient research into the realities of attendants' daily lives and their contribution to asylum care. Melling and Forsythe, *The Politics of Madness*, p. 55.
47. York, 'Alienists, Attendants and the Containment of Suicide'.
48. Wright, *Mental Disability in Victorian England*, p. 99.
49. Ibid.
50. *Asylum News, Journal of the Asylum Workers Association*, 1 (January 1897), p. 4.
51. Scull, *The Most Solitary of Afflictions*. See also K. Jones, *A History of the Mental Health Services* (London, Routledge and Kegan Paul, 1972); K. Jones, *Asylums and After: A Revised History of the Mental Health Services: From the Early Eighteenth Century to the 1900s* (London: Athlone, 1993).
52. Digby, *Madness, Morality and Medicine*, pp. 140–70; Smith, 'Cure, Comfort and Safe Custody', pp. 131–59; D. Wright, 'The Dregs of Society? Occupational Patterns of Male Asylum Attendants in Victorian England', *International History of Nursing Journal*, 1:4 (Summer 1996), pp. 5–19.
53. M. Carpenter, 'Asylum Nursing Before 1914: A Chapter in the History of Labour', in C. Davies (ed.), *Rewriting Nursing History* (London: Croom Helm, 1980), pp. 123–46, on p. 131.
54. Wright, *Mental Disability in Victorian England*, p. 119; MacKenzie, *Psychiatry for the Rich*, p. 144.

55. Rates were similar at other asylums; at Lancaster County Asylum in 1887, male attendants were paid £42–£48 per year, and females received £22–£26. Carpenter, 'Asylum Nursing Before 1914', p. 131.

56. Holloway Annual Report 1899, SHC Acc. 2620/1/1, p. 161. At the private asylum, Ticehurst, wages were described as comparing favourably to those offered for domestic service.

57. P. Nolan, 'A History of the Training of Asylum Nurses', *Journal of Advanced Nursing*, 18 (1993), pp. 1193–201.

58. L. A. Monk, *Attending Madness: At Work in the Australian Colonial Asylum* (Amsterdam: Rodopi, 2008), p. 221.

59. Medico-Psychological Association, *Handbook for the Instruction of Attendants on the Insane* (Boston MA: Cupples, Upham, 1886), p. 122.

60. This is in keeping with findings from other asylums, such as at Kent County. N. Hervey, 'A Slavish Bowing Down: The Lunacy Commission and the Psychiatric Profession 1845–60', in W. F. Bynum, R. Porter and M. Shepherd (eds), *The Anatomy of Madness: Essays in the History of Psychiatry, Vol. 2: Institutions and Society* (London: Routledge Keegan & Paul, 1985), pp. 98–131; Wright, *Mental Disability in Victorian England*, p. 113.

61. Wright, 'The Dregs of Society?', p. 9.

62. The attributes of staff were frequently discussed in the pages of the Annual Reports of the Superintendent.

63. Brookwood Asylum, Miscellaneous Letters and Papers, 1867–1951, uncatalogued and assorted patient's letters, SHC Acc. 6277/PL66, fol. 55.

64. Brookwood Register of Attendants and Servants, SHC Acc. 1523/2/2/1.

65. Brookwood, Miscellaneous Letters and Papers, 1867–1951, uncatalogued and assorted patient's letters, SHC Acc. 6277/PL66, fol. 55.

66. Ibid.

67. Ibid., fol. 67. Neither of these women was successful in their applications. Dr Brushfield may have known the second applicant as he had previously been at Chester for many years.

68. Brookwood, SHC Acc. 3043/Box 36/Bundle 6/31.

69. Holloway Annual Report 1890, SHC Acc. 2620/1/1, p. 40.

70. Holloway Annual Report 1889, WLM28 BE5H74, p. 41.

71. Ibid., p. 23.

72. Holloway Meeting of the General Committee, 17 February 1896, SHC Acc. 2620/1/1, p. 122.

73. Holloway, File of correspondence relating to staff D–F, 1884–1936, SHC Acc. 2620/5/8.

74. Wright, *Mental Disability in Victorian England*, p. 109. At the nearby Earlswood Asylum, the employment of married couples was an overtly acceptable policy from 1874 onwards, although married women accounted for a small percentage of the staff.

75. Brookwood Register of Attendants and Servants, SHC Acc. 1523/2/2/1.

76. Brookwood Reports of the Commissioners in Lunacy 1886, SHC Acc. 1523/1/20, p. 61. At Exminster, half of the female attendants had been employed for less than two years in the 1880s. Melling and Forsythe, *The Politics of Madness*, p. 58.

77. Holloway Annual Report 1899, SHC Acc. 2620/1/1, p. 161. The loss of male attendants referred to does not include the fourteen male reservists serving in the Boer War.

78. Wright, *Mental Disability in Victorian England*, p. 110.

79. Brookwood Register of Attendants and Servants, SHC Acc. 1523/2/2/1, p. 115.

80. Holloway Annual Report 1889, SHC Acc. 2620/1/1, p. 41.

81. Brookwood Register of Attendants and Servants, SHC Acc. 1523/2/2/1.

82. Meeting of the General Committee, 25 February 1900, SHC Acc. 2620/1/1.

83. Rutherford, 'Landscapers for the Mind'. Lloyd's name occurs in connection with at least seven asylum sites and established a reputation in asylum design. He had considerable experience countrywide and was responsible for laying out the garden's at Cane Hill, designed by Howell, Brookwood's architect.

84. Nolan, 'A History of the Training of Asylum Nurses'. Catherine Allen, first Matron at the Retreat, married the Head Attendant George Jepson, and they ran the Retreat until 1823. Dr and Mrs William Ellis worked together at Hanwell from 1831.

85. At the Devon County Asylum, for example, the average day was reported as comprising thirteen hours with only one rest day per fortnight. Melling and Forsythe, *The Politics of Madness*, p. 57.

86. For example, the 1887 Annual Report shows approximately half of all female patients and two-thirds of all male patients were working in Brookwood. SHC Acc. 1523/1/1/6, pp. 52–3.

87. Melling and Forsythe, *The Politics of Madness*, p. 55.

88. Ibid., p. 56. By 1880, this had dropped to fourteen patients per attendant on each side.

89. Brookwood Annual Report 1887, SHC Acc. 1523/1/1/5, p. 60.

90. Holloway Annual Report 1896, SHC Acc. 2620/1/1, p. 126.

91. This was reported to be four male patients to one attendant and five female patients to one nurse; see Melling and Forsythe, *The Politics of Madness*, p. 194.

92. Digby, *Madness, Morality and Medicine*, p. 145; she observes that, in 1877, it stood at 1:5.7. Ticehurst, 1877, employed 150 servants and attendants and 12 companions to care for 63 patients. MacKenzie, *Psychiatry for the Rich*, p. 137. Whilst this amalgamation of categories makes it difficult to assess accurately, Wright for example, concluded that the ratio was less than one patient per attendant.

93. These are discussed in Chapter 4 and 5.

94. Holloway Annual Report 1896, SHC Acc. 2620/1/1, p. 126.

95. Holloway Annual Report 1889, WLM28 BE5H74, p. 11. Failure to comply with legal requirements had seriously delayed Holloway's opening.

96. Medico-Psychological Association, *Handbook for Attendants on the Insane* (London: Baillière, Tindall and Cox, 1899), p. 118.

97. Brookwood Annual Report 1885, SHC Acc. 1523/1/1/3, p. 28.

98. Medico-Psychological Association, *Handbook for Attendants on the Insane*, p. 124.

99. Brookwood Register of Officers and Attendants, SHC Acc. 1523/2/2/1, p. 263.

100. Brookwood Annual Report 1885, SHC Acc. 1523/1/1/3, p. 32.

101. Ibid.

102. Brookwood Annual Report 1893, SHC Acc. 1523/1/2/4, p. 17.

103. Brookwood Report from the Commissioners in Lunacy 1893, SHC Acc. 1523/1/2/4, p. 55.

104. Holloway Annual Report 1887, SHC Acc. 2620/1/1, p. 20.

105. Ibid.

106. Brookwood Register of Officers and Attendants SHC Acc. 1523/2/2/1, p. 225.

107. Brookwood Register of Officers and Attendants, SHC Acc. 1523/2/2/1, p. 1. An extra £3 per year for male attendants and £2 for females was granted in lieu of this.

108. N. McCrae, 'The Beer Ration in Victorian Asylums', *History of Psychiatry*, 155:2 (June 2004), pp. 155–75, on p. 155.
109. Brookwood Register of Officers and Attendants, SHC Acc. 1523/2/2/1, p. 1.
110. Ibid.
111. Brookwood Asylum, Minutes of Committee of Visitors, SHC Acc. 1523/1/9/1, p. 39.
112. Brookwood Asylum, Minutes of Committee of Visitors, Minutes of the Proceedings 15 November 1872 to 17 March 1876, SHC Acc. 1523/1/9/2, 15 May 1874.
113. Brookwood Reports of the Commissioners in Lunacy 1886, SHC Acc. 1523/1/20, p. 61.
114. Brookwood Register of Officers and Attendant, SHC Acc. 1523/2/2/1.
115. The 21st Annual Report of the Committee of Visitors of the Surrey County Lunatic Asylum at Brookwood, 3 April 1888, SHC Acc. 1523/1/1/5.
116. Holloway Annual Report 1889, SHC Acc. 2620/1/1, p. 40.
117. Brookwood Register of Officers and Attendants, SHC Acc. 1523/2/2/1, p. 37.
118. Brookwood, Miscellaneous Letters and Papers, 1867–1951, not catalogued, SHC Acc. 6277/PL66, Bundle 69, letter dated 2 September 1869.
119. Brookwood Female Case Book, SHC Acc. 1523/3/21/1.
120. Brookwood Register of Officers and Attendants, SHC Acc. 1523/2/2/1.
121. Brookwood Register of Officers and Attendants, SHC Acc. 1523/2/2/1, p. 225.
122. Chapter 6 has full details and a discussion of suicide management within the asylums.
123. The 64-page *Handbook* initially received a mixed reception, with some members of the medical profession questioning its value. However, by 1902, it had sold 15,000 copies and was regularly updated. Nolan, 'A History of the Training of Asylum Nurses', p. 1198.
124. Ibid.
125. AWA was apparently inspired by two medical officers and 'Superintendent of Nurses' from Northampton County Asylum, and was intended to include asylum workers of all ranks. M. Arton, 'The Rise and Fall of the Asylum Worker's Association: The History of a Company Union', *International History of Nursing Journal*, 7:3 (Spring 2003), pp. 41–9, on p. 41.
126. *Asylum News, Journal for the Asylum Workers Association*, 1 (January 1897), p. 2.
127. Arton, 'The Rise and Fall of the Asylum Worker's Association', p. 43. As Arton points out, the AWA was formed against a more general background of trade union unrest and so the doctors were opposed to any trade unionism in their institutions, and were keen to offer an alternative association that 'looked after' their workers' interests.
128. *Lancet* (26 December 1896), p. 13.
129. *Asylum News*, 2 (May 1897), p. 6.
130. *Asylum News*, 1 (January 1897), p. 6.
131. Holloway Annual Reports 1895 and 1896, SHC Acc. 2620/1/1. This compares favourably with Exminster Asylum which had twenty-nine male and twenty female attendants holding the certificate by 1903. Melling and Forsythe, *The Politics of Madness*, p. 58.
132. *Asylum News*, 2 (May 1897), p. 6. She was also advised to approach Dr Greene, of Berrywood Asylum, Northampton, although there were 'other Institutions fulfilling the conditions'.
133. Report of the House Committee 1901, General Committee Meetings, SHC Acc. 2620/1/1, p. 184.
134. Holloway Annual Report 1889, SHC Acc. 2620/1/1, p. 41.

135. Interestingly, Kyles was succeeded by one half of another husband and wife team. J. J. Robertson, in addition to becoming Head Attendant, also supervised the outdoor staff whilst his wife became the Housekeeper.
136. Companions were usually only found in expensive private asylums, such as Ticehurst Asylum. By December 1877, there were reportedly twelve male and female companions. MacKenzie, *Psychiatry for the Rich*, p. 137.
137. Holloway Annual Report 1888, SHC Acc. 2620/1/1, p. 26.
138. Holloway Minutes of the General Committee, SHC Acc. 2620/1/1, p. 10.
139. Holloway Annual Report 1888, SHC Acc. 2620/1/1, p. 29.
140. Holloway Miscellaneous, SHC Acc. 2620/5/8, letter dated 18 May 1894.
141. Ibid.
142. Brookwood Register of Officers and Attendants, SHC Acc. 1523/2/2/1, p. 1.
143. Holloway Annual Report 1887, SHC Acc. 2620/1/1, p. 20.
144. Holloway Annual General Meeting, 8 February 1889, Report of the House Committee to the General Committee of the Governors, SHC Acc. 2620/1/1, p. 26.
145. Holloway Annual Report 1888, SHC Acc. 2620/1/1, p. 20.
146. Wright, *Mental Disability in Victorian England*, p. 119.
147. Suicide rates and the treatment of suicidal behaviour in both institutions is the focus of Chapter 6.

3 Origins and Journeys: The Patients at Brookwood Asylum and Holloway Sanatorium

1. The patients' mental diseases are discussed in more detail in Chapter 4.
2. Suicidal behaviour was regarded as a prime indicator of severe mental illness. See Chapter 6.
3. Chancery lunatics were found insane by inquisition which was a procedure where the family and friends of wealthy lunatics petitioned the Lord Chancellor to hold an inquiry so as to prevent the demise of the patient's fortune. A *writ de lunatic inquirrendo* could then be issued and the case heard before a jury. If the verdict of lunacy was upheld, the estate passed to the protection of the Crown. If a compromise was reached pre-trial, then relatives might become involved in the administration of the patient's property.
4. Melling and Forsythe, *The Politics of Madness*, p. 154.
5. D. Wright, 'Delusions of Gender? Lay Identification and Clinical Diagnosis of Insanity in Victorian England', in Andrews and Digby (eds), *Sex and Seclusion*, pp. 149–76, on pp. 157, 174; P. McCandless, 'A House of Cure: The Antebellum South Carolina Lunatic Asylum', *Bulletin of the History of Medicine*, 44 (1990), pp. 220–42, on p. 224.
6. Bartlett, *The Poor Law of Lunacy*, p. 195.
7. Wright, 'Delusions of Gender?', p. 158.
8. R. Adair, W. F. Forsythe and J. Melling, 'A Danger to the Public? Disposing of Pauper Lunatics in Late-Victorian and Edwardian England: Plympton St Mary Union and the Devon County Asylum, 1867–1914', *Medical History*, 42 (1998), pp. 1–25, on p. 11. There is a variance in that the authors state that up to 62 per cent of patients went through the asylum but only 36 per cent gave the workhouse as their previous abode.
9. It fell to 28 and 21 per cent respectively when patients were redistributed due to boundary changes. In this particular year, 175 patients (44 per cent of all admissions) were transferred from Cane Hill Asylum.

10. Brookwood Annual Report 1897, SHC Acc. 1523/2/7, p. 9.
11. Brookwood Annual Report 1900, SHC Acc. 1523/2/10, p. 54.
12. Bartlett, *The Poor Law of Lunacy*, p. 154.
13. Brookwood Female Case Book, SHC Acc. 1523/3/21/18.
14. Ibid.
15. Brookwood Asylum, Report for the Quarter Sessions, 15 October 1867, Minutes of Committee of Visitors, 1867–8, SHC Acc. 1523/1/9/1.
16. Report of the Workhouse Accommodation Committee to the Guildford Board of Guardians 1861.
17. After several years, CLU were obliged to submit to the Corporation of the City of London and the Home Office, and in 1867, many of their harmless lunatics were transferred to the new asylum at Stone, near Dartford, Kent. A. Tanner, 'The City of London Poor Law Union 1837–1869' (PhD dissertation, Birkbeck, University of London, 1995), pp. 218–22.
18. Brookwood Annual Report 1869, SHC Acc. 1523/1/1/1, p. 18.
19. Brookwood Annual Report 1871, SHC Acc. 1523/1/1/2, p. 17.
20. Brookwood Annual Report 1869, SHC Acc. 1523/1/1/1, p. 18.
21. Brookwood Patients Letters and Miscellaneous documents, SHC Acc. 6277, letter dated 17 December 1867.
22. H. Marland, 'Language and Landscapes of Emotion: Motherhood and Puerperal Insanity in the Nineteenth Century', in F. Bound (ed.), *Medicine, Emotion and Disease, 1700–1950* (Basingstoke: Palgrave Macmillan, 2006), pp. 53–77, on p. 60.
23. Brookwood Female Case Book, SHC Acc. 3043/5/9/2/1.
24. Miscellaneous Letters, SHC Acc. 3043/Box 36/2/39. The letter itself is not dated – the date is given by the asylum as the date of receipt.
25. Brookwood Female Case Book, SCH 3043/5/9/1/7.
26. His notes show that only once was he seen to be openly craving alcohol during his stay. Brookwood Male Case Book, SHC 3043/5/9/1/8.
27. Nineteenth-century surgeons were viewed as skilled craftsmen as they were apprenticed, as opposed to physicians, who were generally university educated, so that it was arguably easier and less costly to become a surgeon than a physician. Surgeons' earning capacity was less than that of physicians, so surgeons often doubled as drugs dispensers.
28. A. Tompkins, 'Mad Doctors? The Significance of Medical Practitioners Admitted as Patients to the First English County Asylums up to 1890', *History of Psychiatry*, 23:437 (2012), pp. 437–53, on p. 438.
29. Letter attached in Brookwood Male Case Book, ref: 3043/5/9/1/8, p 219. Underlining as per original.
30. Her fortunes did improve; by 1891 she was Head Matron at Barnardo's Home in Mare Street, Hackney. In 1901, she was the matron (as Katherine Harriet) of the Female institution at 200 Euston Road.
31. By 1881, Henry James was traced as being an inmate at Leavesden Pauper Asylum. Opened in 1870, it was a large Metropolitan Asylums Board (MAB) institution for 'harmless pauper lunatics' from North of the Thames. There was no trace of him in the 1891 census.
32. Tompkins, 'Mad Doctors?', p. 450.
33. Criminal lunatics covered two categories; HMP (Her Majesty's Pleasure) lunatics were those found insane at the time of their trial; and Secretary of State Lunatics were prison-

ers found to be insane during their sentence. HMP lunatics were usually only placed in county asylums if judged to be non-violent.

34. Criminals judged to be insane were often treated more leniently, and could be allowed to complete their sentences within county or borough asylums, particularly if the crime was relatively minor. See Andrews et al., *The History of Bethlem*, pp. 502–3. Following the Criminal Lunatics Act 1884, the Home Secretary was required to consider each HMP case every three years with a view to possible discharge.

35. Broadmoor Criminal Lunatic Asylum was only approximately nine miles from Brookwood. It opened in 1863 and received its first female patients on 27 May and the first male on 27 February 1864. M. Stevens, *Broadmoor Revealed: Victorian Crime and the Lunatic Asylum* (Smashwords edn, 2011); available at www.berkshirerecordoffice.org.uk/albums/broadmoor [accessed 18 December 2013].

36. Brookwood Female Case Book, SHC Acc. 1523/2/21/3.

37. S. Haynes, *Voluntary Patients in Asylums* (Lewes: G. P. Bacon, 1869), p. 3. Stanley Haynes was superintendent of Laverstock House Asylum, near Salisbury. A mixed-class asylum until 1852, it then catered exclusively for the middle classes. There was accommodation for forty-one male and forty-one female patients.

38. Ibid., p. 11.

39. Melling, 'Sex and Sensibility', p. 199.

40. Digby, *Madness, Morality and Medicine*, p. 186.

41. Chancery Lunatics were subject to the supervision of their person and estate by the Masters in Lunacy from 1842. Their lands and/or possessions were given over to the 'committees', frequently next of kin, for the duration of their lunacy. Committal to an asylum was a separate medical procedure.

42. The After-Care Association is discussed in more detail in Chapter 4.

43. *Manchester Courier and Lancashire General Advertiser*, Saturday 22 October 1881, http://www.britishnewspaperarchive.co.uk/viewer/bl/0000206/18811022/097/0011?_=1349623063201 [accessed 7 October 2012].

44. *Morning Post*, 8 November 1862, Naval and Military Intelligence recorded his promotion to first class assistant engineer.

45. Holloway Annual Report 1887, SHC Acc. 2620/1/1, p. 18.

46. Holloway Annual Report 1890, SHC Acc. 2620/1/1, p. 48.

47. Letters may not have been kept for any length of time in deference to perceived middle-class sensibility, or perhaps were lost with the eventual demise of the Holloway Sanatorium nearly a century later when it closed in December 1980.

48. Holloway Male Case Book, SHC Acc. 2620/4/1, pp. 271–2.

49. C. Coleborne, '"His Brain Was Wrong, His Mind Astray", Families and the Language of Insanity, Queensland, and New Zealand, 1880s–1910', *Journal of Family History*, 31:1 (2006), pp. 45–65, on p. 48.

50. Holloway Male Case Book, SHC Acc. 2620/4/1, pp. 271–2.

51. Unfortunately, the case book containing the details of the elder sister, Winifred H.D., and her admissions during 1898 is missing.

52. Holloway Female Case Book, SHC Acc. 3473/5/5.

53. Holloway Register 1885–1892, SHC Acc. 3237/5/1; 1892–1895, SHC Acc. 3237/5/2; 1896–1899, SHC Acc. 3237/5/3.

54. MacKenzie, *Psychiatry for the Rich*, p. 159.

55. Holloway Female Case Book, SHC Acc. 3473/3/1.

56. Incomplete records have survived from Holloway Sanatorium. Origins of the patients have been extrapolated from Holloway Admissions Register 1885–90, containing incomplete data on 281 male and female patients. SHC Acc. 3237/5/1.

57. Holloway Female Case Book, SHC AC 3473/3/5, p. 87.

58. Ibid.

59. Established in 1879 by Reverend Henry Hawkins (of Hanwell Asylum), and initially named the After-Care Association for Poor and Friendless Female Convalescents on leaving Asylums for the Insane. This was amended after men were included from 1894. It is not clear when it changed, but from 1898 the charity was referred to as the After-Care Association for Poor Persons Discharged from Asylums for the Insane. *Bedford Standard*, 25 March 1898.

60. V. Long, 'Changing Public Representations of Mental Illness in Britain 1870–1970' (PhD dissertation, University of Warwick, 2004), p. 191.

61. Annual Report of the Council for the After-Care Association, 1891–92, Wellcome Trust, Contemporary Medical Archives, SA/MAC/B.1/5.

62. R. Hunter and I. Macalpine, *Psychiatry for the Poor: 1851 Colney Hatch Asylum – Friern Hospital 1973* (London: Dawsons of Pall Mall, 1974), p. 207.

63. GPI is discussed further in Chapter 5.

64. Smith, *'Cure, Comfort and Safe Custody'*, p. 108.

65. Brookwood Annual Report 1888, SHC Acc. 1523/1/1/6, p. 26.

66. Brookwood Annual Report 1868, SHC Acc. 1523/1/1/1, p. 16.

67. Brookwood Annual Report 1884, SHC Acc. 1523/1/1/2 p. 23.

68. Brookwood Admissions Registers, 1871, 1881, 1891, SHC Acc. 1523/3/3/1–15.

69. They were also noted in the individual case notes. Causes of insanity for both Brookwood and Holloway patients are discussed more fully in Chapter 4.

70. Brookwood Admissions Registers, 1871–91, SHC Acc. 1523/3/3/1–15.

71. Holloway Admissions Register, 1885–95, SHC Acc. 3237/5/1–2.

72. Brookwood Annual Report 1871, SHC Acc. 1523/1/1/2, pp. 21–4. A second strain that occurred at the same time was attributed to an outbreak of the disease in the local community with which a female attendant had come into contact. In total, twenty-nine were afflicted and five deaths occurred.

73. Holloway did of course have outbreaks of illness, such as influenza in 1891, but nothing on the scale seen at Brookwood.

74. Brookwood Annual Report 1871, SHC Acc. 1523/1/1/2, p. 26.

75. See Chapter 4 for more detail.

76. More discussion of this can be found in Chapter 4.

77. Melling and Forsythe, *The Politics of Madness*, p. 64.

78. Shepherd and Wright, 'Madness, Suicide and the Victorian Asylum', pp. 194–5.

79. Brookwood Annual Report 1871, SHC Acc. 1523/1/1/2, p. 19.

80. According to the 1895 Medical Register, early on in his medical career, Rees Phillips had been engaged as Physician at the Cheltenham Dispensary for Children (established since 1817) and then went on to become a House Surgeon at the Belgrave Hospital for Children, which originally opened in Pimlico in 1866.

81. Brookwood Annual Report 1869, SHC Acc. 1523/1/1/1, p. 23.

82. J. Melling, R. Adair and W. F. Forsythe, '"A Proper Lunatic for Two Years": Pauper Lunatic Children in Victorian and Edwardian England. Child Admissions to the Devon County Asylum, 1845–1914', *Journal of Social History* (Winter 1997), pp. 371–405, on

p. 371. This does not include the monographs on institutions solely dedicated to caring for children, such as Wright's work on the Earlswood Asylum.

83. Ibid., pp. 375, 391.
84. K. Gingell, 'The Forgotten Children: Children Admitted to a County Asylum between 1854 and 1900', *Psychiatric Bulletin*, 25 (2001), pp. 432–4.
85. C. J. Wardle, 'Historical Influences on Services for Children and Adolescents before 1900', in G. Berrios and H. Freeman, *150 Years of British Psychiatry 1841–1991* (London: Athlone Press, 1991), pp. 279–93, on p. 283.
86. Brookwood Annual Report 1869, SHC Acc. 1523/1/1/1, p. 23.
87. Data collected from the Brookwood admissions registers for the census years of 1871, 1881 and 1891, SHC Acc. 1523/3/3/1–15.
88. Data collected from the Brookwood admissions registers for the census years of 1871, 1881 and 1891, SHC Acc. 1523/3/3/1–15.
89. Brookwood Female Casebook, SHC Acc. 3043/5/9/2/7, p. 36.
90. Brookwood Miscellaneous Letters, SHC Acc. 3043, Box 36/2/103.
91. Darenth Asylum for 'imbeciles and school for imbecile children' was erected in 1878 by the managers of the Metropolitan Asylum district (Metropolitan Asylums Board), and was one of the largest establishments of its kind.
92. A. Digby, *Making a Medical Living: Doctors and Patients in the English Market for Medicine, 1720–1911* (Cambridge: Cambridge University Press, 1994), p. 284.
93. Wardle, 'Historical Influences on Services for Children and Adolescents before 1900', p. 283.
94. J. F Beach, 'Insanity in Children', *Journal of Mental Science*, 48 (1898), pp. 459–74, cited in Wardle, 'Historical Influences on Services for Children and Adolescents before 1900', p. 289.
95. Brookwood Female Case Book, SHC Acc. 1523/2/21/3.
96. Brookwood Female Case Book, SHC Acc. 1523/3/21/13.
97. Brookwood Male Case Book, SHC Acc. 1523/3/20/12.
98. Ibid.
99. Brookwood Male Case Book, SHC Acc. 1523/3/20/1.
100. Digby, *Making a Medical Living*, p. 285.
101. Brookwood Annual Report 1884, SHC Acc. 1523/1/1/2, p. 26.
102. Brookwood Annual Report 1895, SHC Acc. 1523/1/2/5, p. 15.
103. Brookwood Annual Report 1897, SHC Acc. 1523/1/2/7, p. 58.
104. The MAB asylums Caterham and Leavesden housed 'imbecile' adults and children, although the children were moved to a temporary smallpox and fever hospital from 1873, before being accommodated at Darenth, Kent, from 1878.
105. Wright, *Mental Disability in Victorian England*, p. 168.
106. Holloway Female Case Book, SHC Acc. 3473/3/5, p. 267.
107. H. Maudsley, *Mind and Body* (London: Macmillan & Co., 1873) cited in Ray, 'Models of Madness', p. 245.
108. The patients' mental diseases are discussed in more detail in Chapter 4.
109. Their varied interactions with the medical profession are further evident in the following chapters on therapeutics and suicidal patients.
110. These slowly evolved, and later legislation regarding defective children would formalize such institutions in the early years of the twentieth century, although their effectiveness was later called into question.

4 'Hurry, Worry, Annoyance and Needless Trouble': Patients in Residence

1. Michael, 'Class, Gender and Insanity in Nineteenth Century Wales', p. 97.
2. Showalter, *The Female Malady*. Some works that questioned the appropriateness of Showalter's analysis include: Andrews and Digby (eds), *Sex and Seclusion*; Ernst, 'European Madness and Gender in Nineteenth-Century British India'; Melling, 'Accommodating Madness'; Smith, *'Cure, Comfort and Safe Custody'*; MacKenzie, *Psychiatry for the Rich*; Wright, 'Getting Out of the Asylum'.
3. Walsh, 'A Class Apart?', pp. 250–1.
4. Ibid., p. 264.
5. Melling and Forsythe, *The Politics of Madness*, p. 149.
6. Brookwood Admissions Registers, SHC, Acc. 1523/3/1/1–15.
7. Brookwood Annual Report 1878, SHC, open shelves, p. 27.
8. Brookwood Annual Report 1871, SHC. Acc. 1523/1/1, p. 19.
9. Shepherd and Wright, 'Madness, Suicide and the Victorian Asylum', p. 183.
10. Melling and Forsythe, *The Politics of Madness*, p. 127; Bartlett, *The Poor Law of Lunacy*, p. 153.
11. P. McCandless, 'A Female Malady? Women at the South Carolina Lunatic Asylum, 1828–1915', *Journal of the History of Medicine and Allied Sciences*, 54 (1999), pp. 543–71, on p. 554.
12. Brookwood's figures taken from Admissions Registers 1867–1906, SHC Acc. 1523/3/1/1–15.
13. Brookwood Annual Report 1871, SHC Acc. 1523/1/1/2, p. 36. In England and Wales, per 1,000 males, there were 1,056 females.
14. Brookwood Annual Report 1871, SHC Acc. 1523/1/1, p. 20.
15. Ibid.
16. These dates were census years, selected as additional documentary evidence could be more easily traced if required.
17. P. Thane, 'Women and the Poor Law In Victorian and Edwardian England', *History Workshop Journal*, 6 (1978), pp. 29–51, on p. 32.
18. Ibid., p. 33.
19. Driver, *Power and Pauperism*, p. 106.
20. These were sparsely furnished, with barred windows and doors that could be locked as required. It is probable that overcrowding, and some allegedly severe cases, led to the managerial, rather than the medical, decision to apply to transfer certain pauper lunatics.
21. The Commissioners in Lunacy frequently adopted a contradictory stance regarding workhouse care of the insane. Bartlett, *The Poor Law of Lunacy*, pp. 44–5.
22. Marland, 'Language and Landscapes of Emotion', p. 73. See also, Marland, *Dangerous Motherhood*.
23. Brookwood Female Case Book, SHC Acc. 1523/3/21/7.
24. These are elaborated later and in the following chapters.
25. This includes both certified patients and voluntary patients.
26. Melling, 'Sex and Sensibility', p. 200.
27. Holloway Annual Report 1891, SHC Acc. 2620/1/1, p. 60.
28. Holloway Annual Report 1890, SHC Acc. 2620/1/1, p. 15.
29. Brookwood Annual Report, 1871, SHC Acc. 1523/1/1/2, p. 20.

30. Sarah. R., Brookwood Female Case Book, SHC Acc. 1523/2/21/3. Two years after her admission, Sarah died in Brookwood. GPI was given as her cause of death.

31. This also includes patients whose records did not have any occupation or remarks recorded in the relevant section of the admissions registers. Census years were again used, as these are the years that comprehensive data was collected from the records to enable easier comparisons elsewhere.

32. There were more than one hundred separate occupations listed in the admissions registers. It was decided to aggregate these into social class categories to make analysis more reliable. The social classification is based on the occupational titles taken from the admissions registers. Details of the Historical International Standard Classification of Occupations (HISCO) can be found at http://historyofwork.iisg.nl/index.php [accessed 30 July 2009].

33. MacKenzie, *Psychiatry for the Rich*, pp. 135–6.

34. Brookwood, from the Patients Admissions Register 1871, SHC Acc. 1523/3/1/5.

35. Brookwood Annual Report 1890, SHC Acc. 1523/1/2/2, p. 13.

36. E. Higgs, *Making Sense of the Census: The Manuscript Returns for England and Wales 1801–1900* (London: HMSO, 1989), p. 99.

37. Often seasonal employment and economic frailty meant that women would turn to prostitution, but this would not have been recorded as a primary occupation. Ballet dancer was another profession that was represented in the admission registers; the term was often synonymous with prostitution and some dancers were obliged to supplement their meagre earnings in this way.

38. Brookwood Female Case Book, SHC Acc. 1523/3/21/7.

39. Melling, 'Sex and Sensibility', p. 186. One retired school mistress and one music teacher was admitted to Brookwood during these years.

40. B. Hill, *Women Alone, Spinsters in England 1600–1850* (New Haven, CT, and London: Yale University Press, 2001), p. 56.

41. Holloway Annual Report 1892, SHC Acc. 2620/1/1, p. 72.

42. Holloway Alphabetical Register of Female Patients, SHC Acc. 3473/3/37.

43. A total of 14,949,624 women as opposed to 14,052,901 men.

44. J. Tosh, *A Man's Place: Masculinity and the Middle Class Home in Victorian England* (New Haven, CT, and London, Yale University Press, 1999), p. 130.

45. Ibid., pp. 152–3.

46. MacKenzie, *Psychiatry for the Rich*, p. 116.

47. Holloway Female Case Book, SHC Acc. 3473/3/3.

48. Ibid.

49. Brookwood Pathological Register, SHC Acc. 3043/4/22.

50. Holloway Female Case Book, SHC Acc. 3473/3/3.

51. Melling and Forsythe, *The Politics of Madness*, p. 137.

52. Holloway Male Casebook, SHC Acc. 3473/3/19.

53. Robert C. registered on 1 January 1859. He was a Licentiate of the Society of Apothecaries in 1852, and MRCSE in 1852.

54. Holloway Male Casebook, SHC Acc. 3473/3/19.

55. Regulations for the Holloway Sanatorium 1886, SHC Acc. 2620.

56. 'The Holloway Sanatorium', pp. 23–4.

57. Holloway Annual Report 1894, SHC Acc. 2620/1/1/2, p. 100.

58. For the years 1885, 1889, 1890 and 1894, the admission data is incomplete and there is no breakdown of males/females available.

59. This strategy was used for many years at other hospitals, including Bethlem. The admission of voluntary patients was established in 1853 and extended to registered hospitals in 1879, Andrews et al., *The History of Bethlem*, p. 654.
60. Holloway Annual Report 1891, SHC Acc. 2620/1/1, p. 59.
61. Holloway Female Case Books, SHC Acc. 3473/3/1, 6, 7, 29.
62. The Coppice opened in 1859, and initially housed sixty first- and second-class patients, as defined by Sneinton Asylum, where overcrowding prompted the building of the Coppice for private and charitable patients. It was closed in the 1980s.
63. Holloway Female Case Book, SHC Acc. 3473/3/1, p. 96.
64. Andrews et al., *The History of Bethlem*; MacKenzie, *Psychiatry for the Rich*, p. 97.
65. MacKenzie, *Psychiatry for the Rich*, p. 136.
66. Brookwood Annual Report 1892, SHC, open shelves, p. 12.
67. Ray, 'Models of Madness', p. 33.
68. Ibid., p. 258.
69. Brookwood Annual Report 1892, SHC, open shelves, p. 12.
70. Brookwood Annual Report 1897, SHC, open shelves, p. 12.
71. Brookwood Annual Report 1899, SHC, open shelves, p. 12. This was 114 patients, calculated against 260 admissions that year. By this date the asylum contained 1088 patients.
72. Melling and Forsythe, *The Politics of Madness*, p. 192.
73. Ibid., p. 202.
74. Brookwood Annual Report 1890, SHC Acc. 1523/1/2/2, p. 22. See also Annual Report for 1896, p. 4.
75. Michael, 'Class, Gender and Insanity in Nineteenth-Century Wales', p. 100.
76. Marland, *Dangerous Motherhood*, p. 165.
77. Thane, 'Women and the Poor Law', p. 34.
78. Marland, *Dangerous Motherhood*, p. 165.
79. Brookwood Annual Report 1871, SHC Acc. 1523/1/1/2, p. 37.
80. Ibid.
81. Brookwood Annual Report 1869, SHC Acc. 1523/1/1/1, p. 24.
82. Brookwood Annual Report 1890, Reports of the County Council, SHC, open shelves, p. 24.
83. This remained the case until 1914. Thane, 'Women and the Poor Law', p. 33.
84. Ibid., pp. 39–40.
85. Brookwood Male Case Book, SHC Acc. 1523/3/20/1.
86. Brookwood Annual Report 1898, SHC, open shelves, p. 11.
87. Holloway Annual Report 1887, SHC Acc. 2620/1/1, p. 19.
88. Ibid.
89. Holloway Annual Report 1895, SHC Acc. 2620/1/1, pp. 113–14.
90. Brookwood Annual Report 1895, SHC Acc. 1523/1/2/5, p. 13. The death rate that year was explained by deaths occurring from influenza and pulmonary disease.
91. 'The Holloway Sanatorium', probably written by George Godwin.
92. Certified patients only.
93. Holloway Annual Report 1887, SHC Acc. 2620/1/1, p. 18.
94. Holloway Annual Report 1900, SHC Acc. 2620/1/1/1, p. 173.
95. Holloway Annual Report 1891, SHC Acc. 2620/1/1, p. 60.
96. Holloway Annual Report 1893, SHC Acc. 2620/1/1, p. 88.
97. Holloway Annual Report 1886, SHC Acc. 2620/1/1, p. 9.
98. Holloway Annual Report 1896, SHC Acc. 2620/1/1, p. 123.

99. Wright, 'Getting Out of the Asylum', pp. 143–4.
100. Ray, 'Models of Madness', p. 234.

5 The Taxonomy and Treatment of Insanity

1. Smith, *'Cure, Comfort and Safe Custody'*, p. 187.
2. Melling and Forsythe, *The Politics of Madness*, p. 61.
3. Wright, *Mental Disability in Victorian England*, p. 24.
4. Ray, 'Models of Madness', *European Journal of Sociology*, p. 237.
5. Ibid., pp. 241–3.
6. S. Tuke, *Description of the Retreat at York* (York: Peirce Isaac, 1815), p .208; cited in Ray, 'Models of Madness', p. 245.
7. Ibid., p. 245.
8. Scull, *Museums of Madness*, especially ch. 6.
9. Patients were removed to a room but not left alone. The superintendent's approach is explained later in the chapter.
10. Digby, *Madness, Morality and Medicine*, p. 123.
11. G. B. Risse and J. H. Warner, 'Reconstructing Clinical Activities: Patient Records', *Social History of Medicine*, 5 (1992), pp. 183–205, on p. 187.
12. T. Claye Shaw, 'Surgical Treatment of General Paralysis of the Insane. Read in the Section of Psychology at the Annual Meeting of the British Medical Association, held in Bournemouth, July 1891', *British Medical Journal* (12 September 1891), pp. 581–3.
13. For example, see G. E. Berrios, 'Of Mania, Introduction', *History of Psychiatry*, 15:1 (2004), pp. 105–24; G. E. Berrios, 'Melancholia and Depression during the Nineteenth Century', *British Journal of Psychiatry*, 153 (1988), pp. 298–304.
14. J. A. B. Tuke, 'A Plea for the Scientific Study of Insanity', *British Medical Journal*, 1 (30 May 1891), pp. 1161–6, on p. 1162.
15. G. E. Berrios, '"Depressive Pseudodementia" or "Melancholic Dementia": A Nineteenth-Century View', *Journal of Neurology, Neurosurgery, and Psychiatry*, 48 (1985), pp. 393–400.
16. Much of the data from the certificates was partially replicated in patient case notes when they were admitted.
17. Wright, 'Delusions of Gender?', pp. 152–3.
18. Chapter 6 discusses the numbers of allegedly suicidal patients admitted in the nineteenth century.
19. Granville, *Care and Cure of the Insane*, for a discussion on this, vol. 2, pp. 156–60.
20. Smith, *'Cure, Comfort and Safe Custody'*, p. 179.
21. Holloway Annual Report 1890, SHC Acc. 2620/1/1, p. 49.
22. As before, the information for Brookwood is taken from the extensive data collected from the census years of 1871, 1881 and 1891; the information for Holloway is taken from 1885 to 1890 due to the limitations of the surviving records.
23. Holloway Annual Report 1888, WLM28 BE5H74, p. 33.
24. Melling and Forsythe, *The Politics of Madness*, p. 195.
25. Brookwood Annual Report 1875, SHC Acc. 1523/1/1/3, p. 18.
26. Melling and Forsythe, *The Politics of Madness*, p. 195.
27. Annual Report of the Visiting Committee of the Surrey County Lunatic Asylum at Brookwood, 21 April 1891, SHC, Reports of the County Council, open shelves, p. 30.
28. Brookwood Male Case Book, SHC Acc. 1523/3/20/5, p. 271.

29. Brookwood Annual Report 1895, SHC Acc. 1523/1/2/5, p. 11.
30. Holloway Annual Report 1890, SHC Acc. 2620/1/1, p. 48.
31. Ibid.
32. Holloway Annual Report 1896, SHC Acc. 2620/1/1, p. 123.
33. Andrews et al., *The History of Bethlem*, cited in Smith, 'Cure, Comfort and Safe Custody', pp. 188, 150–1, 270–6.
34. Granville, *Care and Cure of the Insane*, vol. 2, p. 149.
35. Ibid.
36. Melling and Forsythe, *The Politics of Madness*, pp. 48–9.
37. Granville, *Care and Cure of the Insane*, vol. 1, p. 17.
38. H. Richardson (ed.), *English Hospitals 1660–1948: A Survey of their Architecture and Design* (London: Royal Commission on the Historical Monuments of England, 1998), p. 175.
39. Granville, *Care and Cure of the Insane*, vol. 2, p. 179.
40. Ray, 'Models of Madness', p. 245.
41. Granville, *Care and Cure of the Insane*.
42. Rutherford, 'Landscapers for the Mind', p. 2.
43. Initially, many of Holloway's staff lived off the premises.
44. Holloway Female Case Book, SHC Acc. 3473/3/1. Chapter 6 has full details of this case.
45. Granville, *Care and Cure of the Insane*, vol. 2, pp. 164–7.
46. Ibid., p. 227. Brushfield endorsed the opinion of Dr Cleaton, Rainhill's Medical Superintendent, see p. 180 of the 8 Report of the Commissioners in Lunacy.
47. Brookwood Annual Report 1870, SHC Acc. 1523/1/1/4, p. 6.
48. Nolan, 'A History of the Training of Asylum Nurses', p. 1199.
49. Twenty-eight men were working outside, four in the kitchen and stores, two in the laundry and one in the dining hall and the carpenter's shop. Holloway Annual Report 1888, WLM28 BE5H74, p. 11.
50. Holloway Annual Report 1890, WLM28 BE5H74, p. 10.
51. Brookwood Annual Report 1871, SHC Acc. 1523/1/1/5, p. 28.
52. *Surrey Advertiser*, 1 May 1875, Brookwood SHC Acc. 6277/40.
53. Savage, 'Obituary: Thomas Brushfield'.
54. Ibid.
55. *Surrey Advertiser*, April 1875, precise date unknown, in Brookwood SHC Acc. 6277/40.
56. Anon., 'Fancy-Dress Ball at a Lunatic Asylum', *Illustrated London News* (22 January 1881), p. 86.
57. Ibid.
58. He was Thomas Holloway's brother-in-law. Papers of George Martin Holloway, Royal Holloway Archives, GB131/11/1.
59. At Ticehurst, there was more emphasis on diet, exercise and purging than on hydrotherapy. MacKenzie, 'Social Factors in the Admission', p. 154.
60. Holloway, Annual Report 1896, SHC Acc. 2620/1/1, p. 124.
61. Holloway Annual Report, 1895, SHC Acc. 2620/1/1, p. 113.
62. Holloway Annual Report, 1887, SHC Acc. 2620/1/1, p. 21. By 1888, there was enough room for seven horses and ten carriages.
63. *St Ann's Magazine*, (Christmas 1896), SHC Acc. 2620/6/23.
64. Holloway Annual Report 1899, SHC Acc. 2620/1/2, p. 5.
65. Ibid.

66. Holloway, Rules for the Admission of Patients 1886, SHC Acc. 2620/6/11.
67. This was sold in 1909 to be replaced by purpose built 40-bed accommodation on a 13-acre site at Canford Cliffs in Bournemouth. SHC Acc. 2620, unlisted documents.
68. Holloway Female Voluntary Boarders Case Book, SHC Acc. 3473/3/28.
69. Holloway Annual Report 1887, SHC Acc. 2620/1/1.
70. In both asylums, long-term patients were relegated to specific case books for chronic cases.
71. Brookwood Female Case Book, 3043/5/9/2/3.
72. Brookwood Female Case Book, 1523/3/21/4.
73. Quoted by Brushfield from an 1873 circular issued by the Scottish Commissioners in Lunacy in their seventeenth report. Granville, *Care and Cure of the Insane*, vol. 2, p. 227.
74. Granville, *Care and Cure of the Insane*, vol. 2, p. 225. Brushfield does not say whether the opium treatment was continued once she was admitted to Brookwood.
75. Ibid., p. 226.
76. Holloway Annual Report 1889, WLM28 BE5H74, p. 17.
77. Ibid.
78. Holloway Annual Report 1888, WLM28 BE5H74, p. 11.
79. Holloway Annual Report 1890, WLM28 BE5H74, p. 10.
80. Holloway Female Case Book, SHC Acc. 3473/3/6.
81. 'Report of the Lunacy Commissioners, 26 October 1894', in *Return of the Report of Inquiry Ordered by the Secretary of State for the Home Department into the Causes of Death of a Patient Named Thomas Weir, at St Ann's Heath, Virginia Water, Held by Mr Gully, QC Assisted by Dr George H. Savage* (London, 1895) (Author's own copy), p. 3.
82. On 30 April 2007 this case was included in a Wellcome Seminar by Akinobu Takabayashi, as part of his PhD on psychiatric stigma in twentieth-century Britain.
83. Letters from Mr J. G. Weir, 18 and 25 September 1895 (author's own – to be deposited at SHC). See also *Truth*, 7 March 1895.
84. Holloway, Report of the House Committee 18 February 1895, Meeting of the General Committee 17 February 1896, SHC Acc. 2620/1/1.
85. Weir Mitchell praised its usefulness for treating his private neurasthenia patients in the 1880s. Oppenheim, *'Shattered Nerves'*, p. 120.
86. This is explored further in the chapter devoted to suicide in the asylum.
87. Brookwood Female Case Book, SHC Acc. 1523/3/21/15. Agnes, admitted July 1893, was described as both suicidal and dangerous; she was discharged as recovered in February 1894.
88. Turkish baths were installed in a variety of public and private asylums in the nineteenth century, including Denbeigh, Claybury, Colney Hatch and The Retreat.
89. Eating disorders encompassed many different types of food-associated behaviours, but self-starvation had been recognized for centuries and was often associated with saints and religious figures. Anorexia nervosa became a recognized clinical syndrome in 1873. Brumberg, *Fasting Girls*, pp. 141–53.
90. Holloway Female Case Book, SHC Acc. 3473/3/1.
91. Ibid.
92. Ussher, *Women's Madness*, p. 78.
93. Digby, *Madness, Morality and Medicine*, p. 128.
94. MacKenzie, *Psychiatry for the Rich*, p. 185.
95. Brookwood Male Case Book, SHC Acc. 1523/3/20/1.
96. Chapter 5 provides a detailed examination of this important category of patients.

97. Shepherd and Wright, 'Madness, Suicide and the Victorian Asylum'.

98. Holloway Annual Report 1894, SHC Acc. 2620/1/1, pp. 100–1.

99. Although many of the chemicals that were used are now known to be ineffective or worse, and were unlikely to cure, they were administered at the time in accordance with contemporary medical practice and in the belief that they would possibly do so. The reality is that they may have relieved symptoms and/or produced more biddable patients.

100. Granville, *Care and Cure of the Insane*, vol. 1, p. 59.

101. Opium, of course, provides effective symptom relief.

102. Granville, *Care and Cure of the Insane*, vol. 1, p. 59.

103. Ibid.

104. Brookwood Female Case Book, SHC Acc. 1523/2/21/1, p. 3.

105. Trepanning is one of the oldest known surgical procedures. The operation was used to relieve inflammation, for example from a blow to the head, but it was not a usual procedure carried out in asylums to relieve mental symptoms or GPI, and Brookwood's operation received a great deal of attention in the contemporary medical press.

106. Surgical treatment of GPI was unusual and somewhat controversial under any circumstances; a similar operation had been carried out in 1889 at St Bartholomew's Hospital and subsequently stimulated much debate in the *British Medical Journal*. Claye Shaw, 'The Surgical Treatment of General Paralysis', p. 1090.

107. Brookwood Female Case Book, SHC Acc. 1523/3/21/13. This case stimulated the interest of the medical profession, as indicated by later correspondence between the Brookwood and Banstead Asylum doctors. There are no records of surgical procedures such as this being carried out at the Sanatorium. In August 1892, Augusta was admitted to Wandsworth Asylum as an epileptic, and she died there later that year.

108. Holloway Night Attendant's Report, 1893–7, SHC Acc. 2620/4/3. It is not always clear for whom these prescriptions were intended, as the drugs that were dispensed to both patients and staff were recorded in the same ledger.

109. Holloway Drug Book, November 1894–July 1896, SHC Acc. 3473/4/45.

110. Ibid.

111. V. Berridge, *Opium and the People* (London and New York: St. Martin's Press, Allen Lane, 1981).

112. Digby, *Madness, Morality and Medicine*, p. 127, citing J. C. Bucknill and D. H. Tuke, *A Manual of Psychological Medicine: Containing the History, Nosology, Description, Statistics, Diagnosis, Pathology, and Treatment of Insanity. With an Appendix of Cases* (London: J. and A. Churchill, 1879), p. 477.

113. Holloway Drug Book November 1894–July 1896, SHC Acc. 3473/4/45.

114. I am grateful to Dr H. Allison for his review of drug therapy, March 2000, care of SHC.

115. Adair, Forsythe and Melling, 'A Danger to the Public?', p. 12.

116. SHC Acc. 1523/1/1/3, p. 42. Note the original figures do not tally.

117. This table is reproduced exactly as per the original, miscalculation included. SHC Acc. 1523/1/1/3, p. 42.

118. D. Wright, 'The Discharge of Pauper Lunatics from County Asylums in Mid-Victorian England: The Case of Buckinghamshire', in J. Melling and W. Forsythe (eds.), *Insanity, Institutions and Society 1800–1914* (London: Routledge 1999), pp. 93–112, on pp. 100–3.

119. Ray, 'Models of Madness', p. 229.

120. G. Davis, 'The Most Deadly Disease of Asylumdom: General Paralysis of the Insane and Scottish Psychiatry, c. 1840–1940', *Journal of the Royal College of Physicians*, 42 (Edin-

burgh, 2012), pp. 266–73, on p. 266. See also G. Davis, *'The Cruel Madness of Love': Sex, Syphilis and Psychiatry in Scotland, 1880–1930* (Amsterdam and New York: Rodopi, 2008).

121. Davis, 'The Most Deadly Disease of Asylomdom', p. 270.

122. Nineteenth-century definitions of GPI were broad and inclusive, perhaps partly explaining the variety of symptoms and occasional 'recoveries'. G. Davies, 'The Cruel Madness of Love: Syphilis as a Psychiatric Disorder, Glasgow Royal Asylum 1900–1930' (MPhil dissertation, University of Glasgow, 1997), on p. 11.

123. Brookwood Report of the Superintendent 1875, quoted in Granville, *The Care and Cure of the Insane*, vol. 2, p. 229. During the period 1867–74, there were 279 male deaths of which 126 were GPI (153 were from other causes). There were 172 female deaths, of which only 15 were attributed to GPI (158 were from other causes).

124. 'Report on Brookwood Asylum', *Lancet*, 2 (4 December 1875), p. 817.

125. Brookwood Annual Report 1890, in Surrey County Council Reports 1891, SHC, open shelves, p. 9.

126. Holloway Annual Report 1887, SHC Acc. 2620/1/1, p. 23.

127. Holloway Annual Report 1890, SHC Acc. 2620/1/1, p. 60.

128. Syphilis and GPI were thought of as independent diseases, although in 1886 Thomas Clouston listed syphilis as one of the predisposing causes of GPI. MacKenzie, Social Factors in the Admission', p. 158.

129. Holloway Annual Report 1890, SHC Acc. 2620/1/1, p. 14.

130. This 'league table' is utilized here to illustrate the sanatorium's perception of itself and its competitiveness so that a discussion of admissions is not relevant at this point.

6 Suicide, Self-Harm and Madness in the Asylum

1. G. Berrios and R. Porter (eds), *A History of Clinical Psychiatry: The Origin and History of Psychiatric Disorders* (London: Athlone Press, 1996), pp. 612–32.

2. S. York, 'Suicide, Lunacy and the Asylum in Nineteenth-Century England' (PhD dissertation, University of Birmingham, 2010).

3. It is not the intention to look at the historiography outside of England in this chapter. For a discussion on Durkheim's influence within American psychiatry, see H. I. Kushner, 'American Psychiatry and the Cause of Suicide, 1844–1917', *Bulletin History of Medicine*, 60 (1986), pp. 36–57.

4. M. MacDonald and T. R. Murphy, *Sleepless Souls: Suicide in Early Modern England* (New York: Oxford University Press, 1990); M. MacDonald, 'The Secularization of Suicide in England, 1660–1800', *Past and Present*, 111 (1986), pp. 50–100.

5. MacDonald and Murphy, *Sleepless Souls*.

6. Anderson, *Suicide in Victorian and Edwardian England*.

7. Ibid., esp. ch. 11.

8. B. T. Gates, *Victorian Suicide: Mad Crimes and Sad Histories* (Princeton, NJ: Princeton University Press, 1988).

9. P. Jalland, *Death in the Victorian Family* (Oxford: Oxford University Press, 1996).

10. Prior to 1832, suicides were denied religious ceremony and consecrated ground, although some were discreetly buried in remote sections of churchyards.

11. E. Durkheim, *Le suicide: étude de sociologie* (Paris: Presses universitaires de France, 1897).

12. H. Kushner, 'Suicide, Gender and the Fear of Modernity', in Weaver and Wright (eds), *Histories of Suicide*, pp. 19–52, on p. 20.

13. V. Bailey, *'This Rash Act': Suicide across the Life Cycle in the Victorian City* (Stanford, CA: Stanford University Press, 1998).

14. Shepherd and Wright, 'Madness, Suicide and the Victorian Asylum'.

15. S. York, 'The Asylum and Suicide Prevention in the Age of Non-Restraint' (MA dissertation, Oxford Brookes University, 2003).

16. York, 'Alienists, Attendants and the Containment of Suicide'.

17. W. W. Westcott, *Suicide Its History, Literature, Jurisprudence, Causation, and Prevention. A Social Science Treatise* (London: H. K. Lewis, 1885), p. 126.

18. G. H. Savage, 'Constant Watching of Suicidal Cases', *Journal of Mental Science*, 30 (1884), pp. 17–19, on p. 17.

19. 25 & 26 Vict. c. 111, s. 44.

20. Morselli was Professor of Psychological Medicine at Royal University Turin, and Chief Physician to the Royal Asylum for the Insane.

21. Savage, 'Constant Watching of Suicidal Cases'; Westcott, *Suicide Its History*; H. Morselli, *Suicide, an Essay on Comparative Moral Statistics* (London: C. Kegan Paul Co., 1881).

22. It also suggests that the absence of a desire to commit suicide was a central determinant in the decision of medical superintendents to recommend to county magistrates the discharge of patients back into the community.

23. York, 'The Asylum and Suicide Prevention', p. 14.

24. Ibid., pp. 14–15, Digby, *Madness, Morality and Medicine*; S. Cherry, *Mental Health Care in Modern England, The Norfolk Lunatic Asylum/St Andrew's Hospital, 1810–1998* (Woodbridge: Boydell Press, 2003).

25. Parry-Jones, *The Trade In Lunacy*.

26. Digby, *Madness, Morality and Medicine*, pp. 79–80.

27. F. Winslow, *The Anatomy of Suicide* (London: Henry Renshaw, 1840), p. 5.

28. R. Brown, *The Art of Suicide* (London: Reaktion, 2001), p. 147.

29. J. Conolly, *An Inquiry Concerning the Indications of Insanity with Suggestions for the Better Care and Protection of the Insane* (1830; London: J. Taylor, reprint 1973), pp. 256–7.

30. Winslow, *The Anatomy of Suicide*, p. 164.

31. J. Haslam, *Observations on Madness and Melancholy: Including Practical Remarks on Those Diseases; Together with Cases: and an Account of the Morbid Appearances on Dissection* (London: Printed for C. Callow, by G. Hayden 1809), p. 308.

32. Ibid., p. 309.

33. Winslow, *The Anatomy of Suicide*, p. 189.

34. Brushfield, 'On Medical Certificates of Insanity', p. 712.

35. Ibid.

36. Ibid.

37. Westcott, *Suicide Its History*, p. 126. He used 1882 figures from the Reports of the Commissioners in Lunacy for England and Wales.

38. Ibid.

39. A. T. Scull, *The Most Solitary of Afflictions: Madness and Society in Britain, 1700–1900* (New Haven, CT, and London: Yale University Press, 2005), p. 346.

40. Ibid., p. 236.

41. J. C. Bucknill and D. H. Tuke, *A Manual of Psychological Medicine* (London: J. and A. Churchill, 1874), quoted in Westcott, *Suicide Its History*, p. 121.

42. Morselli, *Suicide, an Essay*, p. 197.

43. Gates, *Victorian Suicide*, pp. 125–7. Havelock Ellis (1859–1939) was a social activist, physician and psychologist. He was also a believer in eugenic principles and was the president of the Galton Institute.

44. H. Kushner, 'Suicide, Gender, and the Fear of Modernity in Nineteenth-Century Medical and Social Thought', *Journal of Social History*, 26:3 (Spring 1993), pp. 461–90, on p. 462.

45. Ibid.

46. Winslow, *The Anatomy of Suicide*, quoted in Kushner, 'Suicide, Gender and the Fear of Modernity in Nineteenth-Century Medical and Social Thought', p. 464.

47. Kushner, 'Suicide, Gender and the Fear of Modernity'; T. G. Masaryk, *Suicide and the Meaning of Civilisation* (1881; Chicago, IL: University of Chicago Press, reprinted 1970). Thomas Masaryk (1850–1937) was the future Liberal Democratic founder of Czechoslovakia.

48. Today, amongst those who self-harm, women still dominate, whilst there are more completed suicides amongst men. See Oxford Centre for Suicide Research, at www.cebnh. warne.ox.ac.uk/csr/recentpubs.html.

49. Calculated from Brookwood Registers of Admissions, 1871 and 1881, SHC Acc. 1523/3/1/1–15.

50. Brookwood Annual Report 1878, SHC Acc. 1523/1/1/3, p. 34.

51. Morselli, *Suicide, an Essay*, p. 200. Granville, *The Care and Cure of the Insane*, vol. 2, p. 228.

52. Holloway Female Case Book, SHC Acc. 3473/3/6.

53. Granville, *Care and Cure of the Insane*.

54. Westcott, *Suicide Its History*, p. 146.

55. Ibid.

56. Adapted from Westcott's combined estimates for suicides in 1881 and 1882. Westcott, *Suicide Its History*, p. 147, W. Ogle, 'Suicides in England and Wales in Relation to Age, Sex, Season and Occupation', *Journal of the Royal Statistical Society* (March 1886), pp. 101–35, on p. 118, table 9.

57. Brookwood Male Case Book, SHC Acc. 1523/3/20/2.

58. Brookwood Male Case Book, SHC Acc. 3043/5/9/1/8. After a fairly non-eventful time in Brookwood during which he worked in the tailor's shop, George was discharged as recovered on 16 July 1878.

59. Shepherd and Wright, 'Madness, Suicide and the Victorian Asylum'.

60. Patients who deliberately harm themselves have a risk of suicide some 100 times greater than that of the general population. See for example, E. Murphy et al., 'Risk Factors for Repetition and Suicide Following Self-Harm in Older Adults: Multicentre Cohort Study', *British Journal of Psychiatry*, 200:5 (May 2012), pp. 399–404. The risk of suicide was 67 times that of older adults in the general population.

61. S. Chaney, 'Self-Control, Selfishness and Mutilation: How 'Medical' is Self-Injury Anyway?', *Medical History*, 55:3 (July 2011), pp. 375–82.

62. Brookwood Female Case Book, SHC Acc. 1523/3/21/6.

63. Ibid.

64. Brookwood Annual Report 1893, SHC Acc. 1523/1/2/4, p. 17.

65. Brookwood Male Case Book, SHC Acc. 1523/3/20/13.

66. Ibid.

67. Medico-Psychological Association, *Handbook for Attendants on the Insane*, p. 126.

68. Brushfield, 'On Medical Certificates of Insanity', p. 712.

69. Holloway Annual Report 1898, SHC Acc. 2620/1/1.
70. Holloway Annual Report 1894, SHC Acc. 2620/1/1.
71. Savage, 'Constant Watching of Suicidal Cases', p. 19.
72. Holloway Annual Report 1894, SHC Acc. 2620/1/1.
73. Ibid.
74. MacKenzie, *Psychiatry for the Rich*, p. 179.
75. Holloway Annual Report 1897, SHC Acc. 2620/1/1.
76. Holloway Annual Report 1891, SHC Acc. 2620/1/1.
77. Holloway Female Case Book, SHC Acc. 3473/3/1.
78. Holloway Female Case Book, SHC Acc. 3473/3/1. This patient remained in Holloway until her death in October 1918.
79. Holloway Female Case Book, SHC Acc. 3473/3/6. Rose was eventually transferred to Peckham House in 1904.
80. Holloway Female Case Book, SHC Acc. 3473/3/28.
81. R. Houston, 'The Medicalization of Suicide: Medicine and the Law in Scotland and England, circa 1750–1850', in Weaver and Wright (eds), *Histories of Suicide*, pp. 91–118.
82. Brookwood Female Case Book, SHC Acc. 1523/3/21/6.
83. Kushner, 'Suicide, Gender and the Fear of Modernity', p. 27.
84. York, 'The Asylum and Suicide Prevention', p. 15.
85. Scull, *The Most Solitary of Afflictions*, p. 300. Scull, however, believed that this ideal of moral treatment was undermined by the dramatic growth of asylums.
86. Westcott, *Suicide Its History*, p. 128.
87. Brookwood Annual Report 1878, SHC Acc. 1523/1/1/3.
88. Holloway Female Case Book, SHC Acc. 3473/3/1.
89. Holloway Annual Report 1894, SHC Acc. 2620/1/1.
90. A. Shepherd, 'The Female Patient Experience in Two Late Nineteenth Century Surrey Asylums', in Andrews and Digby (eds), *Sex and Seclusion*, pp. 223–48.
91. *West Middlesex Herald*, 26 March 1887.
92. Holloway Female Case Book, SHC Acc. 3473/3/1.
93. Brookwood Male Case Book, SHC Acc. 1523/3/20/2.
94. Brookwood Female Case Book, SHC Acc. 1523/3/21/2.
95. At Brookwood, references to galvanization have been traced in 1893, as detailed in Chapter 5.
96. Holloway Female Case Book, SHC Acc. 3473/3/1.
97. Brookwood Female Case Book, SHC Acc. 1523/3/21/2.
98. It is has not been possible to ascertain what it was at Springfield that so agitated this patient. Her completed suicide may be partially attributed to the large numbers of inmates, negating effective surveillance.
99. 'Thirty-Sixth Report of the Commissioners in Lunacy, 31 March 1882' *Parliamentary Papers* (PP), 1882, vol. 32, pp. 89, 98–112, 199.
100. H. F. H. Newington, 'What are the Tests of Fitness for Discharge from Asylums?', *Journal of Mental Science*, 32 (1886–7), pp. 491–500.
101. Digby, *Madness, Morality and Medicine*, p. 199.
102. MacKenzie, *Psychiatry for the Rich*, p. 179.
103. Brookwood Male Case Book, SHC Acc. 1523/3/20/4.
104. Holloway Male Case Book, SHC Acc. 3473/3/21.
105. Anderson, *Suicide in Victorian and Edwardian England*, p. 403. From 0.63 per cent in 1867 to 0.14 per cent in 1911.

106. Digby, *Madness, Morality and Medicine*, p. 198.

107. Anderson, *Suicide in Victorian and Edwardian England*, pp. 377–81.

108. Westcott, *Suicide Its History*, p. 119.

109. This could mean care by a relative or friend, either at home or in a similar environment, or the patient could be cared for within the unlicensed house of a medical or layman. The Commissioners in Lunacy were able, but not obliged, to visit these patients, and magistrates had no powers of inspection or jurisdiction. D. Bower, 'The Means at Present Provided by Law for the Care and Cure of Non-Pauper Lunatics, and its Safeguards', *British Medical Journal* (30 July 1881), pp. 152–3. (Bowers was MD of Springfield House Asylum, Bedford.)

110. Anderson, *Suicide in Victorian and Edwardian England*, p. 103; Westcott, *Suicide Its History*, p. 108.

111. Ibid., p. 94.

Conclusion

1.   Wright, 'The Discharge of Pauper Lunatics from County Asylums in Mid-Victorian England'.

2.   Ray, 'Models of Madness'.

3.   Showalter, *The Female Malady*.

4.   Melling, Adair and Forsythe, 'A Proper Lunatic for Two Years'.

5.   Holloway Sanatorium did slowly adopt selective aspects of what would now be termed occupational therapy, but these were less rigorously implemented than at the public asylum.

6.   Anderson, *Suicide in Victorian and Edwardian England*.

WORKS CITED

Manuscripts

Brookwood Asylum, Report of the Workhouse Accommodation Committee to the Guild-ford Board of Guardians, 1860, Surrey History Centre (hereafter SHC), Acc. 6277/70.

—, Robert Rawlinson, Report on the Proposed Site of Surrey Asylum, 13 May 1861, National Archives, MH83/260.

—, First Annual Report of Brookwood Asylum for 1867, Wellcome Library for the History of Medicine Archives (hereafter WLM) WLM28 BE5 S96.

—, C. H. Howell, Report on the Surrey Asylum, 16 March 1868, National Archives, MH83/260.

—, Admissions Registers, 1867–1906, Acc. 1523/3/1/1–15.

—, Annual Reports of Committee of Visitors of Surrey County Lunatic Asylum at Brook-wood, to Quarter Sessions, 1884–8, SHC Acc. 1523/1/1/1–6.

—, Annual Report of the Visiting Committee of the Surrey County Lunatic Asylum at Brookwood, 21 April 1891, SHC, Reports of the County Council, open shelves.

—, Case Books, Females, 1867–1896, SHC Acc. 1523/3/21/1–16.

—, Case Books, Males, 1867–1905, SHC Acc. 1523/3/20/1–14.

—, Case Book, Males, 1903–4, SHC Acc. 3043/5/9.

—, General Rules, 1867, 1873, 1879, 1890, SHC Acc.1523/2/1/3–5.

—, *Rules for the Guidance of Attendants and Servants and All Persons Engaged in the Service of the Surrey County Asylum at Brookwood*, 1871, SHC Acc. 1523/2/1/1.

—, Register of Officers, Attendants and Servants, 1866–1924, SHC Acc. 1523/2/2/1.

—, Reports of the Medical Superintendent in the Annual Reports of Committee of Visitors of Surrey County Lunatic Asylum at Brookwood, to Quarter Sessions, 1868–88, SHC Acc. 1523/1/1/1–6.

—, Reports of the Medical Superintendent in the Annual Reports of Committee of Visi-tors of Surrey County Lunatic Asylum at Brookwood, to Quarter Sessions, 1890–1908, SHC Acc. 1523/1/2/2–17.

—, Reports of Commissioners in Lunacy to the Lord Chancellor 1868–86, SHC Acc. 1523/9/1–37b.

—, Miscellaneous Letters and Papers, 1867–1951, not catalogued, SHC Acc. 6277/PL66.

—, Surrey Quarter Session: Minutes of Committee of Visitors of Brookwood Asylum, 1867–93, SHC Acc. 1523/1/9/1–6.

—, *Surrey Advertiser*, 1 April 1875, SHC Acc. 6277/40.

—, *Surrey Advertiser*, 1 May 1875, Brookwood SHC Acc. 6277/40.

—, *Surrey Advertiser*, 20 June 1885, SHC Acc. 6277/4/0.

Holloway Sanatorium, Reports of the Medical Superintendent in the Reports for the Administrative County of Surrey, 1891–9, SHC, open shelves.

—, Admissions Register, 1885–95, SHC Acc. 3237/5.

—, Copy of the Hospital Rules for the Admission and Visiting of Patients, 50, contained in the Holloway Annual Report 1888, WLM28 BE5H74.

—, Annual Reports, Holloway Sanatorium, 1888–90, WLM28 BE5H74.

—, Female Case Books, 1885–1910, SHC Acc. 3473/3/1–9.

—, Male Case Books, 1891–1898, SHC Acc. 3473/3/19–21.

—, Female Voluntary Boarders Case Books – 1890–1909, SHC Acc. 3473/3/28–29.

—, Male Voluntary Boarders Case Book – 1897–1907, SHC Acc. 3473/3/33.

—, Case Books, 1889–1926, MSS.5157–63, 8159–60.

—, Alphabetical Register of Female Patients, 1885–1919, SHC Acc. 3473/3/37.

—, Alphabetical Register of Male Patients, 1885–1931, SHC Acc. 3473/3/40.

—, Post-Mortem Book, 1899–1927, SHC Acc. 3473/3/56.

—, Patients Book, 1885–1929, SHC Acc. 3473/3/64.

—, Drug Books, 1894–1900, SHC Acc. 3473/4/45–46.

—, Miscellaneous, SHC Acc. 2620/5/8.

—, Regulations for the Holloway Sanatorium, Hospital for the Insane, St Ann's Heath, Virginia Water, 1886, SHC Acc. 2620.

—, Annual Reports 1886–1906, Minutes of the Annual and Ordinary Meetings of the General Committee for Holloway Sanatorium, SHC Acc. 2620/1/1.

—, Minutes of the House Committee, 31 December 1885–3 May 1892, SHC Acc. 2620/2/1.

—, Night Attendant's Report, 1893–1897, SHC Acc. 2620/4/3.

—, Staff Register, Male, 1895–1935 SHC Acc. 2620/5/1.

—, Staff Register, Female, 1895–1935 SHC Acc. 2620/5/2.

—, Correspondence Relating to Staff, 1897–1939, SHC Acc. 2620/5/7–13.

—, 'Suggestions and Instructions in Reference to a Proposed Lunatic Asylum at St Ann's Heath, near Virginia Water Station, Surrey', Holloway papers, 1872, SHC Acc. 2620/6/1.

—, Correspondence and Papers Relating to Opening Celebrations for the Sanatorium, 1884–5, SHC Acc. 2620/6/2.

—, Charity Commission Deed, 29 January 1889, SHC Acc. 2620/6/5.

—, Regulations for the Holloway Sanatorium Approved by the Secretary of State, 1885–1925, SHC Acc. 2620/6/9.

—, Rules for the Admission, Visiting and Discharge of Patients, 1886, SHC Acc. 2620/6/11.

—, *St Ann's Occasional Magazine*, 33 (Christmas 1896), Holloway Miscellaneous Papers, SHC Acc. 2620/6/23.

—, Annual Report of the Council for the After-Care Association, 1891–92, Wellcome Trust, Contemporary Medical Archives, SA/MAC/B.1/5.

—, Papers of George Martin Holloway, Royal Holloway Archives, GB131/11/1.

Primary Sources

Anon., 'Visiting Physicians to County Asylums', *Asylum Journal*, 1 (1854).

—, 'How to Spend a Quarter of a Million, or More', *Builder*, 29:1468 (25 March 1871), p. 220.

—, 'In What Way Can Good Best be Done?', *Builder*, 29:1470 (8 April 1871), p. 297.

—, 'How Best to Spend Money for the Public Good?', *Builder*, 29:1471 (15 April 1871), pp. 277–9.

—, 'In What Way Can Good Best be Done?', *Builder*, 29:1472 (22 April 1871), pp. 297–8.

—, 'The Competition Designs for Proposed Lunatic Asylums at S. Ann's Heath', *Building News and Engineering Journal*, 23:916 (2 August 1872), pp. 75–7.

—, 'Lunatic Asylum, S. Anne's Heath', *Building News and Engineering Journal*, 23:927 (11 October 1872), p. 282.

—, 'The Holloway Sanatorium, Virginia Water', *Builder*, 25:1797 (14 July 1877), p. 710.

—, 'Fancy-Dress Ball at a Lunatic Asylum', *Illustrated London News* (22 January 1881), p. 86.

—, 'Holloway College and Sanatorium, Virginia Water', *Building News and Engineering Journal*, 41:1393 (16 September 1881), p. 356.

—, 'The Holloway Sanatorium', *Builder*, 43: 2031 (7 January 1882), pp. 23–4.

—, 'An Asylum and an Elysium', *Woman* (31 August 1892).

—, 'The Holloway In-Sanatorium', *Truth*, 37:949 (7 March 1895), pp. 585–7.

—, 'Obituary: Thomas Brushfield', *Lancet* (31 December 1910), p. 2054.

—, 'Obituary: The Late Sir James M. Moody', *British Journal of Psychiatry* (September 1915), p. 519.

—, 'Obituary: Dr Rees Philipps', *British Medical Journal* (23 January 1926), p. 172.

—, Holloway College and Sanatorium Virginia Water', *Building News*, 45 (16 September 1881), pp. 393, 356.

Asylum News, Journal of the Asylum Workers Association, 1 (January 1897), pp. 2, 4; 2 (May 1897), p. 6.

Bartholomew, J., *Gazetteer of the British Isles* (London: A and C Black, 1887).

Bower, D., 'The Means at Present Provided by Law for the Care and Cure of Non-Pauper Lunatics, and its Safeguards', *British Medical Journal*, 2 (30 July 1881), pp. 152–3.

Brushfield, T. N., 'Application of Photography to Lunacy', *Journal of the Photographic Society*, 3 (21 May 1857), p. 289.

—, 'On Medical Certificates of Insanity', *Lancet*, 115:2958 (8 May 1880), pp. 711–3.

—, 'On Medical Certificates of Insanity', *Lancet*, 115:2961 (29 May 1880), pp. 830–2.

—, 'Practical Hints on the Treatment, Symptoms, and Medico-Legal Aspects of Insanity', read before the Chester Medical Society, 1890.

Bucknill, J. C. and D. H. Tuke, *A Manual of Psychological Medicine: Containing the History, Nosology, Description, Statistics, Diagnosis, Pathology, and Treatment of Insanity. With an Appendix of Cases* (London: J. and A. Churchill, 1879).

Claye Shaw, T., 'Surgical Treatment of General Paralysis of the Insane. Read in the Section of Psychology at the Annual Meeting of the British Medical Association, held in Bournemouth, July 1891', *British Medical Journal* (12 September 1891), pp. 581–3.

Conolly, J., *An Inquiry Concerning the Indications of Insanity with Suggestions for the Better Care and Protection of the Insane* (1830; London: John Taylor, reprint 1973).

—, 'Lectures on the Construction and Government of Lunatic Asylums', *Lancet*, 113 (4 July 1846), pp. 2–5.

Dickens, C., 'A Curious Dance around a Curious Tree', *Household Words* (17 January 1852), pp. 387–8.

Dunglison, R., *A Dictionary of Medical Sciences* (Philadelphia, PA: Blanchard and Lea, 1856).

Durkheim, E., *Le suicide: etude de sociologie* (Paris: Presses universitaires de France, 1897).

Granville, J. M., *Care and Cure of the Insane*, 2 vols (London: Hardwicke and Bogue, 1877).

Haslam, J., *Observations on Madness and Melancholy: Including Practical Remarks on Those Diseases; Together with Cases: and an Account of the Morbid Appearances on Dissection* (London: Printed for C. Callow, by G. Hayden, 1809).

Haynes, S., *Voluntary Patients in Asylums* (Lewes: G. P. Bacon, 1869).

Low, S., *The Charities of London* (London: Sampson Low, Son, and Marston, 1867).

Manchester Courier and Lancashire General Advertiser, Saturday 22 October 1881, at http://www.britishnewspaperarchive.co.uk [accessed 7 October 2012].

Masaryk, T. G., *Suicide and the Meaning of Civilisation* (1881; Chicago, IL: Chicago University Press, reprinted 1970).

Medico-Psychological Association, *Handbook for the Instruction of Attendants on the Insane* (Boston, MA: Cupples, Upham, 1886).

—, *Handbook for Attendants on the Insane* (London: Baillière, Tindall and Cox, 1899).

Morning Post, 8 November 1862, at http://www.britishnewspaperarchive.co.uk [accessed 7 October 2012].

Morselli, H., *Suicide, an Essay on Comparative Moral Statistics* (London: C. Kegan Paul Co., 1881).

Newington, H. F. H., 'What are the Tests of Fitness for Discharge from Asylums?' *Journal of Mental Science*, 32 (1886–7), pp. 491–500.

Ogle, W., 'Suicides in England and Wales in Relation to Age, Sex, Season and Occupation', *Journal of the Royal Statistical Society* (March 1886), pp. 101–35.

'Report of the Lancet Commission on Lunatic Asylums: Brookwood Asylum', *Lancet*, 2 (4 December 1875), pp. 816–20.

'Report on Brookwood Asylum', *Lancet*, 2 (4 December 1875), p. 227.

'Report of the Lunacy Commissioners, 26 October 1894', in *Return of the Report of Inquiry Ordered by the Secretary of State for the Home Department into the Causes of Death of a Patient Named Thomas Weir, at St Ann's Heath, Virginia Water, Held by Mr Gully, QC Assisted by Dr George H. Savage* (London, 1895).

Savage, G. H., 'Constant Watching of Suicidal Cases', *Journal of Mental Science*, 30 (1884), pp. 17–19.

—, 'Obituary: Thomas Brushfield', *British Medical Journal* (31 December 1910), p. 2054.

'Thirty-Sixth Report of the Commissioners in Lunacy, 31 March 1882', *Parliamentary Papers* (PP), 1882, vol. 32.

Tuke, J. A. B., 'A Plea for the Scientific Study of Insanity', *British Medical Journal*, 1 (30 May 1891), pp. 1161–6.

Westcott, W. W., *Suicide Its History, Literature, Jurisprudence, Causation, and Prevention* (London: H. K. Lewis, 1885).

Winslow, F., *The Anatomy of Suicide* (London: Henry Renshaw, 1840).

Secondary Sources

Adair, R., W. F. Forsythe and J. Melling, 'A Danger to the Public? Disposing of Pauper Lunatics in Late-Victorian and Edwardian England: Plympton St. Mary Union and the Devon County Asylum, 1867–1914', *Medical History*, 42:1 (1998), pp. 1–25.

Anderson, O., *Suicide in Victorian and Edwardian England* (Oxford: Clarendon Press, 1987).

Andrews, J., A. Briggs, R. Porter, P. Tucker and K. Waddington, *The History of Bethlem* (London: Routledge, 1997).

Andrews, J., 'Case Notes, Case Histories, and Patients' Experience of Insanity at Gartnavel Royal Asylum, Glasgow, in the Nineteenth Century', *Social History of Medicine*, 11 (1998), pp. 255–81.

Andrews, J. and A. Digby (eds), *Sex and Seclusion, Class and Custody: Perspectives on Gender and Class in the History of British and Irish Psychiatry* (Amsterdam and New York: Rodopi, 2004).

Arton, M., 'The Rise and Fall of the Asylum Worker's Association: The History of a Company Union', *International History of Nursing Journal*, 7:3 (Spring 2003), pp. 41–9.

Ayers, G. M., *England's First State Hospitals and the Metropolitan Asylums Board, 1867–1930* (London: Wellcome Institute of the History of Medicine, 1971).

Bailey, V., *'This Rash Act': Suicide across the Life Cycle in the Victorian City* (Stanford, CA: Stanford University Press, 1998).

Bartlett P., 'The Asylum, the Workhouse and the Voices of the Insane Poor in Nineteenth-Century England', *International Journal of Law and Psychiatry*, 21 (1998), pp. 421–32.

—, *The Poor Law of Lunacy: The Administration of Pauper Lunatics in Mid-Nineteenth-Century England* (London: Leicester University Press, 1999).

Bartlett, P. and D. Wright, *Outside the Walls of the Asylum: The History of Care in the Community 1750–2000* (London: Athlone, 1999).

Berridge, V., *Opium and the People* (London and New York: St. Martin's Press, Allen Lane, 1981).

Berrios, G. E., '"Depressive Pseudodementia" or "Melancholic Dementia": A Nineteenth-Century View', *Journal of Neurology, Neurosurgery, and Psychiatry*, 48 (1985), pp. 393–400.

—, 'Melancholia and Depression during the Nineteenth Century', *British Journal of Psychiatry*, 153 (1988), pp. 298–304.

—, *The History of Mental Symptoms: Descriptive Psychopathology since the Nineteenth Century* (Cambridge: Cambridge University Press, 1996).

—, 'Of Mania, Introduction', *History of Psychiatry*, 15:1 (2004), pp. 105–24.

Berrios, G. E. and H. Freeman (eds), *150 Years of British Psychiatry, 1841–1991* (London: Athlone Press, 1991).

— (eds), *150 Years of British Psychiatry: Volume 2: The Aftermath* (London: Athlone Press, 1996).

Berrios, G. and R. Porter (eds), *A History of Clinical Psychiatry: The Origin and History of Psychiatric Disorders* (London: Athlone Press, 1996).

Best, G., *Mid-Victorian Britain 1851–75* (London: Weidenfeld and Nicholson, 1979).

Bound, F. (ed.), *Medicine, Emotion and Disease, 1700–1950* (Basingstoke: Palgrave Macmillan, 2006).

Brown, R., *The Art of Suicide* (London: Reaktion, 2001).

Brumberg, J. J., *Fasting Girls: The Emergence of Anorexia Nervosa as a Modern Disease* (London: Harvard University Press, 1998).

Bynum, W. F., R. Porter and M. Shepherd (eds), *The Anatomy of Madness: Essays in the History of Psychiatry, Volume 2: Institutions and Society* (London: Tavistock, 1985).

Carpenter, M., 'Asylum Nursing Before 1914: A Chapter in the History of Labour', in C. Davies (ed.), *Rewriting Nursing History* (London: Croom Helm, 1980), pp. 123–46.

Chaney, S., 'Self-Control, Selfishness and Mutilation: How "Medical" is Self-Injury Anyway?', *Medical History*, 55:3 (July 2011), pp. 375–82.

Cherry, S., *Mental Health Care in Modern England: The Norfolk Lunatic Asylum and St. Andrew's Hospital, 1810–1998* (Woodbridge: Boydell Press, 2003).

Coleborne, C., 'Families, Patients and Emotions: Asylums for the Insane in Colonial Australia and New Zealand, c. 1880–1910', *Social History of Medicine*, 19 (2006), pp. 425–42.

—, '"His Brain Was Wrong, His Mind Astray", Families and the Language of Insanity, Queensland, and New Zealand, 1880s–1910', *Journal of Family History*, 31:1 (2006), pp. 45–65.

Davis, G., 'The Cruel Madness of Love: Syphilis as a Psychiatric Disorder, Glasgow Royal Asylum 1900–1930' (MPhil dissertation, University of Glasgow, 1997).

—, *'The Cruel Madness of Love': Sex, Syphilis and Psychiatry in Scotland, 1880–1930* (Amsterdam and New York: Rodopi, 2008).

—, 'The Most Deadly Disease of Asylumdom: General Paralysis of the Insane and Scottish Psychiatry, c. 1840–1940', *Journal of the Royal College of Physicians*, 42 (Edinburgh, 2012), pp. 266–73.

Digby, A., *Madness, Morality and Medicine: A Study of the York Retreat, 1796–1914* (Cambridge: Cambridge University Press, 1985).

—, 'Moral Treatment at the Retreat, 1796–1846', in Bynum, Porter and Shepherd (eds), *The Anatomy of Madness: Volume 2: Institutions and Society*, pp. 52–72.

—, *Making a Medical Living: Doctors and Patients in the English Market for Medicine, 1720–1911* (Cambridge: Cambridge University Press, 1994).

Driver, F., *Power and Pauperism: The Workhouse System, 1834–1884* (Cambridge: Cambridge University Press, 1993).

Dwyer, E., *Homes for the Mad: Life inside Two Nineteenth-Century Asylums* (New Brunswick, NJ: Rutgers University Press, 1987).

Dyos, H. J., *Victorian Suburb: A Study of the Growth of Camberwell* (Leicester: Leicester University Press, 1961).

Elliot, J., *Palaces, Patronage and Pills – Thomas Holloway: His Sanatorium, College and Picture Gallery* (Egham: Royal Holloway, 1996).

Ernst, W., 'European Madness and Gender in Nineteenth-Century British India', *Social History of Medicine*, 9:3 (1996), pp. 357–82.

Forsythe, W., J. Melling and R. Adair, 'The New Poor Law and the County Pauper Lunatic Asylum: The Devon Experience 1834–1884', *Social History of Medicine*, 9:3 (December 1996), pp. 335–55.

Foucault, M., *Madness and Civilisation: A History of Insanity in the Age of Reason*, trans. R. Howard (London: Tavistock, 1965).

French, C. N., *The Story of St Luke's Hospital* (London: W. Heinemann, 1951).

Gates, B. T., *Victorian Suicide: Mad Crimes and Sad Histories* (Princeton, NJ: Princeton University Press, 1988).

Gingell, K., 'The Forgotten Children: Children Admitted to a County Asylum between 1854 and 1900', *Psychiatric Bulletin*, 25 (2001), pp. 432–4.

Harrison-Barbet, A., *Thomas Holloway, Victorian Philanthropist* (Egham: Royal Holloway, 1994).

Hervey, N., 'A Slavish Bowing Down: The Lunacy Commission and the Psychiatric Profession 1845–60', in Bynum, Porter and Shepherd (eds), *The Anatomy of Madness: Volume 2: Institutions and Society*, pp. 98–131.

Higgs, E., *Making Sense of the Census: The Manuscript Returns for England and Wales 1801–1900* (London: HMSO, 1989).

Hill, B., *Women Alone, Spinsters in England 1600–1850* (New Haven, CT, and London: Yale University Press, 2001).

Hirst, D. and P. Michael, 'Family, Community and the Lunatic in Mid-Nineteenth-Century North Wales', in Bartlett and Wright (eds), *Outside the Walls of the Asylum*, pp. 66–85.

Houston, R., 'The Medicalization of Suicide: Medicine and the Law in Scotland and England, circa 1750–1850', in Weaver and Wright (eds), *Histories of Suicide*, pp. 91–118.

Hunter, R. and I. Macalpine, *Psychiatry for the Poor: 1851 Colney Hatch Asylum – Friern Hospital 1973* (London: Dawsons of Pall Mall, 1974).

Jalland, P., *Death in the Victorian Family* (Oxford: Oxford University Press, 1996).

Jansson, A., 'Mood Disorders and the Brain: Depression, Melancholia, and the Historiography of Psychiatry', *Medical History*, 55:3 (July 2011), pp. 393–99.

Jones, C. and R. Porter (eds), *Reassessing Foucault: Power, Medicine, and the Body* (London: Routledge, 1994).

Jones, K., *A History of the Mental Health Services* (London: Routledge and Kegan Paul, 1972).

—, *Asylums and After: A Revised History of the Mental Health Services: From the Early 18th Century to the 1990s* (London: Athlone, 1993).

Karthas, I., 'The Politics of Gender and the Revival of Ballet in Early Twentieth Century France', *Journal of Social History*, 45:4 (2012), pp. 960–89.

Kushner, H. I., 'American Psychiatry and the Cause of Suicide, 1844–1917', *Bulletin of the History of Medicine*, 60 (1986), pp. 36–57.

—, 'Suicide, Gender, and the Fear of Modernity in Nineteenth-Century Medical and Social Thought', *Journal of Social History*, 26:3 (Spring 1993), pp. 461–90.

—, 'Suicide, Gender and the Fear of Modernity', in Weaver and Wright (eds), *Histories of Suicide*, pp. 19–52.

Lodge Patch, I., 'The Surrey County Lunatic Asylum (Springfield): Early Years in the Development of an Institution', *British Journal of Psychiatry*, 159 (1991), pp. 69–77.

Long, V., 'Changing Public Representations of Mental Illness in Britain 1870–1970' (PhD dissertation, University of Warwick, 2004.)

McCandless, P., 'A House of Cure: The Antebellum South Carolina Lunatic Asylum', *Bulletin of the History of Medicine*, 44 (1990), pp. 220–42.

—, 'A Female Malady? Women at the South Carolina Lunatic Asylum, 1828–1915', *Journal of the History of Medicine and Allied Sciences*, 54 (1999), pp. 543–71.

McCrae, N., 'The Beer Ration in Victorian Asylums', *History of Psychiatry*, 155:2 (June 2004), pp. 155–75.

MacDonald, M., 'The Secularization of Suicide in England, 1600–1800', *Past and Present*, 111 (1986), pp. 50–100.

MacDonald, M. and T. R. Murphy, *Sleepless Souls: Suicide in Early Modern England* (New York: Oxford University Press, 1990).

MacKenzie, C., 'Social Factors in the Admission, Discharge, and Continuing Stay of Patients at Ticehurst Asylum, 1845–1917', in Bynum, Porter and Shepherd (eds), *The Anatomy of Madness, Volume 2: Institutions and Society*, pp. 147–74.

—, 'The Life of a Human Football: Women and Madness in the Era of the New Woman', *Society for the Social History of Medicine Bulletin* (1985), pp. 37–40.

—, *Psychiatry for the Rich: A History of Ticehurst Private Asylum, 1792–1917* (London and New York: Routledge, 1992).

MacKinnon, D., '"Amusements are Provided": Asylum Entertainment and Recreation in Australia and New Zealand, c. 1860–c. 1945', in G. Mooney and J. Reinarz (eds), *Permeable Walls*, pp. 267–88.

Marland, H., *Dangerous Motherhood: Insanity and Childbirth in Victorian Britain* (London and Basingstoke: Palgrave Macmillan, 2004).

—, 'Language and Landscapes of Emotion: Motherhood and Puerperal Insanity in the Nineteenth Century', in Bound (ed.), *Medicine, Emotion and Disease*, pp. 53–77.

Melling, J., 'Accommodating Madness: New Research in the Social History of Insanity and Institutions', in J. Melling and W. Forsythe (eds), *Insanity, Institutions and Society*, pp. 1–30.

—, 'Sex and Sensibility in Cultural History: The English Governess and the Lunatic Asylum, 1845–1914', in Andrews and Digby (eds), *Sex and Seclusion*, pp. 177–221.

Melling, J., R. Adair and W. F. Forsythe, '"A Proper Lunatic for Two Years": Pauper Lunatic Children in Victorian and Edwardian England. Child Admissions to the Devon County Asylum, 1845–1914', *Journal of Social History* (Winter 1997), pp. 371–405.

Melling, J. and W. Forsythe (eds), *Insanity, Institutions and Society, 1800–1914: A Social History of Madness in Comparative Perspective* (London: Routledge, 1999).

—, *The Politics of Madness, the State, Insanity and Society in England, 1845–1914* (London: Routledge, 2006).

Michael, P., *Care and Treatment of the Mentally Ill in North Wales 1800–2000* (Cardiff: Cardiff University Press, 2000).

—, 'Class, Gender and Insanity in Nineteenth Century Wales', in Andrews and Digby (eds), *Sex and Seclusion*, pp. 95–122.

Monk, L. A., *Attending Madness: At Work in the Australian Colonial Asylum* (Amsterdam: Rodopi, 2008).

Mooney, G. and J. Reinarz (eds), *Permeable Walls: Historical Perspectives on Hospital and Asylum Visiting* (Amsterdam and New York: Rodopi, 2009).

Murphy, E., 'The Lunacy Commissioners and the East London Guardians, 1845–1867', *Medical History*, 46 (2002), pp. 495–524.

Murphy, E., N. Kapur, R. Webb, N. Purandare, K. Hawton, H. Bergen, K. Waters and J. Cooper, 'Risk Factors for Repetition and Suicide Following Self-Harm in Older Adults: Multicentre Cohort Study', *British Journal of Psychiatry*, 200:5 (May 2012), pp. 399–404.

Nolan, P., 'A History of the Training of Asylum Nurses', *Journal of Advanced Nursing*, 18 (1993), pp. 1193–201.

Oppenheim, J., *'Shattered Nerves': Doctors, Patients and Depression in Victorian England* (New York and Oxford: Oxford University Press, 1991).

Oxford Centre for Suicide Research, at www.cebnh.warne.ox.ac.uk/csr/recentpubs.html [accessed 26 May 2011].

Parry-Jones, W. L., *The Trade in Lunacy: A Study of Private Madhouses in England in the Eighteenth and Nineteenth Centuries* (London: Routledge and Kegan Paul, 1972).

—, 'The History of Child and Adolescent Psychiatry: Its Present Day Relevance', *Journal of Child Psychology and Psychiatry*, 30:1 (1989), pp. 3–11.

Patch, I. L., 'The Surrey County Lunatic Asylum (Springfield). Early Years in the Development of an Institution', *British Journal of Psychiatry*, 159 (1991), pp. 69–77.

Philo, C., '"Fit Localities for an Asylum": The Historical Geography of the Nineteenth-Century "Mad Business" in England as Viewed Through the Pages of the Asylum Journal', *Journal of Historical Geography*, 13:4 (1987), pp. 398–415.

Porter, R., *The Social History of Madness* (London: Weidenfield and Nicholson, 1987).

—, *Mind-Forg'd Manacles: A History of Madness in England from the Restoration to the Regency* (London: Athlone, 1987).

Prestwich, P. E., 'Family Strategies and Medical Power: "Voluntary" Committal in a Parisian Asylum, 1876–1914', *Journal of Social History*, 27:4 (June 1994), pp. 797–816.

Ray, L. J., 'Models of Madness in Victorian Asylum Practice', *European Journal of Sociology*, 22 (1981), pp. 229–64.

Renvoize, E., 'The Association of Medical Officers of Asylums and Hospitals for the Insane, the Medico-Psychological Association and their Presidents', in Berrios and Freeman (eds), *150 Years of British Psychiatry 1841–1991*, pp. 29–78.

Richardson, H. (ed.), *English Hospitals 1660–1948: A Survey of their Architecture and Design* (London: Royal Commission on the Historical Monuments of England, 1998).

Risse G. B. and J. H. Warner, 'Reconstructing Clinical Activities: Patient Records', *Social History of Medicine*, 5 (1992), pp. 183–205.

Rutherford, S., 'Landscapers for the Mind: English Asylum Designers, 1845–1914', *Garden History*, 33:1 (Summer 2005), pp. 2–19.

Saint, A., 'Holloway Sanatorium: A Conservation Nightmare', *Victorian Society Annual* (1993), pp. 19–34.

Scull, A. T., *Museums of Madness: The Social Organisation of Insanity in Nineteenth-Century England* (London: Allen Lane, 1979).

— (ed.), *Madhouses, Mad-Doctors, and Madmen: The Social History of Psychiatry in the Victorian Era* (London: Athlone, 1981).

—, *The Most Solitary of Afflictions: Madness and Society in Britain, 1700–1900* (New Haven, CT, and London: Yale University Press, 1993).

—, 'Rethinking the History of Asylumdom', in Melling and Forsythe (eds), *Insanity, Institutions and Society*, pp. 295–315.

—, *The Most Solitary of Afflictions: Madness and Society in Britain, 1700–1900* (New Haven, CT, and London: Yale University Press, 2005).

Scull, A. T., C. MacKenzie and N. Hervey, *Masters of Bedlam: The Transformation of the Mad-Doctoring Trade* (Princeton, NJ: Princeton University Press, 1996).

Shepherd, A., 'The Female Patient Experience in Two Late Nineteenth-Century Surrey Asylums', in Andrews and Digby (eds), *Sex and Seclusion*, pp. 223–48.

Shepherd, A. and D. Wright, 'Madness, Suicide and the Victorian Asylum: Attempted Self-Murder in the Age of Non-Restraint', *Medical History*, 46:2 (April 2002), pp. 175–96.

Showalter, E., *The Female Malady: Women, Madness and English Culture 1830–1980* (London: Virago, 1987).

Smith C., 'Family, Community and the Victorian Asylum: A Case Study of the Northampton General Lunatic Asylum and its Pauper Lunatics', *Family and Community History*, 9:2 (2006), pp. 109–24.

Smith, L. D., *'Cure, Comfort and Safe Custody': Public Lunatic Asylums in Early Nineteenth-Century England* (London: Leicester University Press, 1999).

—, '"Your Very Thankful Inmate": Discovering the Patients of an Early County Lunatic Asylum', *Social History of Medicine*, advanced access, 3 June 2008, at http://shm.oxford-journals.org/cgi/content/full/hkn030v1 [accessed 9 July 2009].

Stevens, M., *Broadmoor Revealed: Victorian Crime and the Lunatic Asylum* (Smashwords edn, 2011); available at www.berkshirerecordoffice.org.uk/albums/broadmoor [accessed 18 December 2013].

Suzuki, A., 'The Politics and Ideology of Non-Restraint: The Case of the Hanwell Asylum', *Medical History*, 39 (1995), pp. 1–17.

—, *Madness at Home: The Psychiatrist, the Patient and the Family in England, 1820–1860* (Berkeley, CA: University of California Press, 2006).

Tanner, A., 'The City of London Poor Law Union 1837–1869' (PhD dissertation, Birkbeck, University of London, 1995).

Taylor, J., *Building for Healthcare: Hospital and Asylum Architecture in England 1840–1914* (London and New York: Mansell, 1991).

—, 'The Architect and the Pauper Asylum in Late Nineteenth-Century England. G. T. Hine's 1901 Review of Asylum Space and Planning', in Topp, Moran and Andrews, *Madness, Architecture and the Built Environment*, pp. 263–84.

Thane, P., 'Women and the Poor Law in Victorian and Edwardian England', *History Workshop Journal*, 6 (1978), pp. 29–51.

Tompkins, A., 'Mad Doctors? The Significance of Medical Practitioners Admitted as Patients to the First English County Asylums up to 1890', *History of Psychiatry*, 23:437 (2012), pp. 437–53.

Topp, L., J. E. Moran and J. Andrews, *Madness, Architecture and the Built Environment: Psychiatric Spaces in Historical Context* (London: Routledge, 2007).

Tosh, J., *A Man's Place: Masculinity and the Middle Class Home in Victorian England* (New Haven, CT, and London: Yale University Press, 1999).

Ussher, J., *Women's Madness: Misogyny or Mental Illness?* (Hemel Hempstead: Harvester Wheatsheaf, 1991).

Vandereycken W. and R. van Deth, 'Who Was the First to Describe Anorexia Nervosa: Gull or Lasègue?' *Psychological Medicine*, 19:4 (November 1989), pp. 837–45.

Walsh, L., 'A Class Apart? Admissions to the Dundee Royal Lunatic Asylum', in Andrews and Digby (eds), *Sex and Seclusion*, pp. 249–70.

Walton, J., *The British Seaside: Holidays and Resorts in the Twentieth Century* (Manchester: Manchester University Press, 2000).

Walton, J. K., 'Casting Out and Bringing Back in Victorian England: Pauper Lunatics, 1840–1870', in Bynum, Porter and Shepherd (eds), *The Anatomy of Madness: Volume 2: Institutions and Society*, pp. 132–46.

Wannell, L., 'Patients' Relatives and Psychiatric Doctors: Letter Writing in the York Retreat, 1875–1910', *Social History of Medicine*, 20:2 (2007), pp. 297–313.

Wardle, C. J., 'Historical Influences on Services for Children and Adolescents before 1900', in Berrios and Freeman (eds), *150 Years of British Psychiatry 1841–1991*, pp. 279–93.

Wright, D., 'The Dregs of Society? Occupational Patterns of Male Asylum Attendants in Victorian England', *International History of Nursing Journal*, 1:4 (Summer 1996), pp. 5–19.

—, 'Getting Out of the Asylum: Understanding the Confinement of the Insane in the Nineteenth Century', *Social History of Medicine*, 10:1 (1997), pp. 137–55.

—, 'The Certification of Insanity in Nineteenth-Century England and Wales', *History of Psychiatry*, 9 (1998), pp. 267–90.

—, 'The Discharge of Pauper Lunatics from County Asylums in Mid-Victorian England: The Case of Buckinghamshire', in J. Melling and W. F. Forsythe (eds), *Insanity, Institutions and Society*, pp. 93–112.

—, 'Asylum Nursing and Institutional Service: A Case Study of the South of England, 1861–1881', *Nursing History Review*, 7 (1999), pp. 153–69.

—, *Mental Disability in Victorian England: The Earlswood Asylum, 1847–1901* (Oxford: Oxford University Press, 2001).

—, 'Delusions of Gender? Lay Identification and Clinical Diagnosis of Insanity in Victorian England', in Andrews and Digby (eds), *Sex and Seclusion*, pp. 149–76.

Weaver J. and D. Wright (eds), *Histories of Suicide: International Perspectives on Self-Destruction in the Modern World* (Toronto: University of Toronto Press, 2009).

York, S., 'The Asylum and Suicide Prevention in the Age of Non-Restraint' (MA dissertation, Oxford Brookes University, 2003).

—, 'Suicide, Lunacy and the Asylum in Nineteenth-Century England' (PhD dissertation, University of Birmingham, 2010).

—, 'Alienists, Attendants and the Containment of Suicide in Public Lunatic Asylums, 1845–1890', *Social History of Medicine*, 25:2 (2012), pp. 324–42.

INDEX